Health Care in World Cities

Health Care in World Cities

New York, Paris, and London

MICHAEL K. GUSMANO, PH.D.
VICTOR G. RODWIN, PH.D., M.P.H.
DANIEL WEISZ, M.D., M.P.A.

The Johns Hopkins University Press

Baltimore

© 2010 The Johns Hopkins University Press
All rights reserved. Published 2010
Printed in the United States of America on acid-free paper
9 8 7 6 5 4 3 2 1

The Johns Hopkins University Press
2715 North Charles Street
Baltimore, Maryland 21218-4363
www.press.jhu.edu

Library of Congress Cataloging-in-Publication Data

Gusmano, Michael K.
  Health care in world cities : New York, Paris, and London / Michael K. Gusmano,
Victor G. Rodwin, and Daniel Weisz.
      p. ; cm.
  Includes bibliographical references and index.
  ISBN-13: 978-0-8018-9444-2 (hardcover : alk. paper)
  ISBN-10: 0-8018-9444-1 (hardcover : alk. paper)
    1. Health status indicators—New York (State)—New York. 2. Health status
indicators—France—Paris. 3. Health status indicators—England—London. 4. Urban
health. I. Rodwin, Victor. II. Weisz, Daniel. III. Title.
    [DNLM: 1. Delivery of Health Care—London. 2. Delivery of Health Care—New
York City. 3. Delivery of Health Care—Paris. 4. Cities—London. 5. Cities—New
York City. 6. Cities—Paris. 7. Cross-Cultural Comparison—London. 8. Cross-Cultural
Comparison—New York City. 9. Cross-Cultural Comparison—Paris.
W 84 AN7 G982h 2010]
RA407.G87 2010
614.4'2421—dc22   2009030726

A catalog record for this book is available from the British Library.

*Special discounts are available for bulk purchases of this book. For more information,
please contact Special Sales at 410-516-6936 or specialsales@press.jhu.edu.*

The Johns Hopkins University Press uses environmentally friendly book materials,
including recycled text paper that is composed of at least 30 percent post-consumer waste,
whenever possible. All of our book papers are acid-free, and our jackets and covers are
printed on paper with recycled content.

CONTENTS

Preface   vii
Acknowledgments   xi

1. A New Approach to Comparing Health Systems   1

2. Comparable Cities within Contrasting Health Systems   21

3. Overall Performance of the Health System:
   Avoidable Mortality   56

4. Access to Primary Care: Avoidable Hospital Conditions   74

5. Access to Specialty Care: The Treatment of Heart Disease   93

6. Conclusions   115

Appendix: Data and Methods   129
References   153
Index   175

New York, Paris, and London are among the largest cities in some of the wealthiest nations of the world. They are strategic locations for transnational corporations, as well as for governments and international organizations. Although they consider themselves unique, these cities share many characteristics and problems. As centers for specialized financial and legal services, media, and culture, they exercise a powerful influence, not only on their own nations, but also on the rest of the world. Their inhabitants are heterogeneous, including some of the wealthiest and poorest members of their respective nations, and they attract the "creative classes" (Florida, 2005) that contribute to innovation and economic growth.

Aside from serving as vast engines of economic growth, world cities are characterized by large and growing disparities in wealth, income, housing, and health. They provide relatively high levels of public services and public transportation, and they attract people from their extensive metropolitan regions—indeed, from around the world—to their universities, museums, theaters, and libraries. As centers for biomedical research and specialized medical care, these cities also provide access to state-of-the-art health services. Many of their hospitals serve as national, even global, centers of excellence, attracting patients worldwide; such hospitals include the Memorial Sloan-Kettering Cancer Center and New York–Presbyterian Medical Center in Manhattan, Hôpital Saint Louis or Hôpital Européen-Georges Pompidou in Paris, and Guy's and St. Thomas's hospitals in London. Alongside such venerable institutions are equally well-known hospitals and health centers that serve the most disadvantaged populations. In New York, a vast network of public hospitals and health centers serves as a safety net for those without health insurance and for a significant share of the Medicaid population. In Paris and London, with their systems of universal coverage, there is not a formal safety net system separate from the public institutions, but special initiatives are targeted to serve the needs of the most vulnerable populations.

Chapter 1 sets the context for our analysis of health system performance by reviewing the literature that compares the health care systems and population health of cities and by presenting a new approach to comparing the health care systems of New York, Paris, and London. Chapter 2 provides an overview of the broader health system context of each nation and the salient features of the health systems and public health infrastructure in each city. We then present the rationale for our systematic comparisons across and within our three cities. Chapters 3, 4, and 5 analyze several dimensions of access to health care based on three indicators: "avoidable mortality," avoidable hospital conditions, and revascularization (coronary artery bypass surgery and angioplasty) adjusted for the burden of disease. Each of these chapters explores aggregate measures of access and disparities within each city and what we define in Chapter 2 as their "urban cores": Manhattan, Paris, and Inner London. (When we refer to policies, practices, and/or empirical findings that apply to the entire city, we refer to New York City and London. When we refer to our empirical findings for the urban cores, we refer to Manhattan and Inner London. For Paris, there is no distinction between the city and the urban core. As we explain in Chapter 2, for Paris, the equivalent of New York City and Greater London is Paris and its three surrounding departments.) The final chapter summarizes the most striking similarities and differences among the health care systems of New York, Paris, and London; reflects on the value of our approach to comparative health systems analysis; and speculates on the lessons drawn from our findings.

Our city-level comparisons produce some evidence that reinforces well-known critiques of our health care system and other evidence that questions the conventional wisdom on health system performance and access to care across these systems. For example, a recent comparison of England and the United States indicates that the English have better health status than Americans (Banks et al., 2006). This has led some journalists to suggest that the National Health Service (NHS) provides better access to health care than the U.S. system.* Our empirical analysis, however, reveals a

---

* In fairness, the authors of the study do not make this claim or support this view—but that has not prevented some members of the media from making this claim.

more complex reality. In Chapter 3, our examination of avoidable mortality indicates that residents of England and of Inner London have higher levels of premature death that, in theory, could have been "avoided" with better access to timely and effective health care than do their counterparts in the United States and Manhattan. If, on average, the English are healthier than Americans, this is probably not due to better access to these health care services. Before we judge the NHS too harshly, however, it is important to note that we do not observe the same magnitude of neighborhood disparities in avoidable mortality in Inner London that we find in Manhattan. Overall, access to health services that reduce avoidable mortality may be greater in Manhattan than in Inner London, but inequality of access to timely and effective health care is greater in Manhattan than in Paris or Inner London. If we place significant weight on equity, it is less clear which of these systems is preferable—a question to which we return in Chapter 6.

In Chapter 4 we present evidence that access to primary care in Manhattan is considerably worse than in Paris or Inner London, where all residents benefit from systems of universal health care coverage. This failure to assure universal access to basic health care services results in high rates of avoidable hospitalizations and a more hospital-centered health care system than Paris or London.

In Chapter 5, however, our findings stand in stark contrast to conventional wisdom on access to revascularization services in the United States compared with that of health systems that provide universal coverage. Although we do not provide health insurance to all of our citizens and there are large gaps in access to health care, we spend more on health care services than any other nation, particularly on invasive procedures. Evidence of this comes from comparisons of revascularization rates among countries of the Organization for Economic Cooperation and Development (OECD). The rate of revascularization is about three times higher in the United States than in the next highest nation and four times higher than the OECD average. We demonstrate, however, that once we account for differences in the burden of heart disease, residents of the United States and Manhattan have lower rates of revascularizations than do their counterparts in France and Paris.

What explains this remarkable finding? Once we account for differences in burden of disease, U.S. patients with private health insurance are receiving revascularizations at about the same rate as residents of Paris and France. Patients in Manhattan and the United States with no health insurance or public insurance (Medicare or Medicaid—or both) have lower rates of revascularizations than residents of Paris and France. In summary, under France's national health insurance program, hospitals and doctors are using surgery to treat heart disease in about the same way that U.S. hospitals and doctors use these procedures for residents with private health insurance. When we examine OECD health data, the United States provides higher rates of revascularizations than most wealthy nations, in part because the burden of heart disease is greater among our residents than among those of most other countries. Despite the higher burden of disease, Manhattan and the United States appear to provide a lower rate of revascularization than Paris and France because large segments of the U.S. population have poor access to these surgical procedures.

As we discuss in more detail in Chapter 6, we are struck by how often health systems abroad with universal coverage are mischaracterized as "government-run" systems that interfere with clinical decision making. In contrast to such caricatures, our analysis sheds light on how two systems providing universal health care coverage—a national health service in London and national health insurance in Paris—operate in practice. An unambiguous conclusion is that, however much these systems are similar in providing universal coverage, they do so with different levels of funding, distinct institutional structures, and contrasting opportunities for access to different levels of care. Finally, our comparisons suggest that although similar places share our problems, the extent of inequalities in access to health care that is evident in Manhattan is not apparent in Paris and Inner London.

ACKNOWLEDGMENTS

This book would not have been possible without extensive contributions from family, friends, and colleagues. Our families have endured our long absences during trips to France and England—and even longer absences due to time spent at the International Longevity Center–USA in Manhattan, where we completed much of the analysis and writing for this book. We thank Katie, Joseph, Allie, Nadell, Leonora, Aaron, and Louise for their love and patience.

Several colleagues helped us complete this work by asking probing questions, making helpful suggestions, and offering encouragement. They are responsible for many of the book's strengths, but we alone are responsible for its limitations. We thank Christa Altenstetter, Volker Amelung, Talley Andrews, Dennis Andrulis, Asheesh Bhalla, Howard Berliner, Emmanuelle Cadot, Pierre Chauvin, Jan Blustein, Aurélie Bocquier, Fréderic Bousquet, Lawrence D. Brown, Rachel Bursac, Mame-Yaa Busumtwi, Paul Corrigan, Dhiman Das, Laurent Degos, Serena Deng, Marc Duriez, Marc Esponda, Francis Fagnani, Oliver Fein, Sherry Glied, Marguerite Grady, Thomas Heil, Bobbie Jacobson, Emily Katz, Anthony Kovner, Karl Kronebusch, Roger Kropf, Olivier Lacoste, Claude LePen, Theodore Marmor, Martin McKee, Jean-Paul Moatti, Véronique Moysan, Harry "Rick" Moody, Charlotte Muller, Ellen Nolte, Yolande Obadia, Kieke Okma, Adam Oliver, Dominique Polton, Len Rodberg, Jean-Louis Salomez, Katie Shea, Diane Slama-Lequet, Michael Sparer, Alfred Spira, Jeanne Stellman, Rosemary Stevens, Frédéric Van Roekeghem, Florence Veber, David Vlahov, Caitlin Warbelow, and Jessica Watterson. In addition, Wendy Harris, our editor at the Johns Hopkins University Press, and two anonymous reviewers encouraged us to refine our analysis and clarify the goals of the book.

We presented early drafts of the chapters of this book at a number of meetings, including seminars at the American University of Paris, Cornell

University, Columbia University, the "Age-Boom" Academy of the ILC-USA, the London School of Economics and Political Science, New York University, and the New York Health Policy Group. We also presented this work at conferences organized by the American Medical Association, the Hong Kong Hospital Authority, the Massachusetts Medical Society, NHS London, and the Observatoire Régionale de la Santé in Lille and Marseille. We thank the participants for their comments and suggestions.

We acknowledge financial support from the Florence V. Gould Foundation, the French Ministry of Health (Direction de l'Hospitalisation et de l'Organisation des Soins), the Health Care Foundation of New Jersey, the Jacob and Valeria Langeloth Foundation, the New York Community Trust, the New York City Department for the Aging, and the R. W. Johnson Health Policy Investigator Award Program. Our special thanks go to Robert N. Butler, Everette Dennis, and the entire staff of the ILC-USA and its board of directors for their generous financial and intellectual support of the World Cities Project (WCP) (www.ilcusa.org/projects).

Finally, we would like to dedicate this book to the memory of our colleague Leland G. Neuberg. Leland was a valued member of the extended WCP team. We are grateful for his friendship and his many efforts to improve the quality of our analysis.

Health Care in World Cities

CHAPTER ONE

A New Approach to Comparing Health Systems

MUCH HAS BEEN WRITTEN about New York, Paris, and London, but comparative studies of these cities are scarce, and those that do exist have not examined the health care systems and population health of these cities. Beyond the temptation of exploring uncharted territory, the most compelling reason for comparing health systems across these world cities is that, in spite of the trumpeted claims by each city as being unique within its own nation, they have much in common and therefore provide a notable opportunity for more refined comparisons and cross-national learning. Given their common characteristics, comparative analyses of their different health care systems can provide insights into the possible effects of national and local policies on such outcomes as the use of services and health status. Surely, it would be imprudent to draw causal inferences from an in-depth comparison of three cases. But the differences we observe can suggest possibilities for mutual learning and promising directions for further research.

Beyond contributing to research, there is a pragmatic and perhaps even more important reason for studying health care in world cities. In the world's megacities—defined by the United Nations as urban agglomerations with more than 10 million inhabitants—policy makers are searching for models of how to organize public health infrastructure and accommodate the growth of urban populations. There are now 26 megacities with populations of more than 10 million people and 40 cities with populations of between 5 and 10 million (UN, 2008). Indeed, the rise of megacities has been called the defining megatrend of the twenty-first century (www.192021.org, accessed July 1, 2008). The experience of world cities in wealthier nations in establishing public health infrastructure, developing health systems, and attempting to overcome their own inequalities among diverse neighborhoods may provide useful lessons in meeting the daunting challenges of megacities in developing nations (Linden, 1996). By comparing world cities in three contrasting national health policy contexts, our analysis provides insights into the effects of national policy on urban health systems and the health of city residents.

Despite the importance of megacities and increasing urbanization worldwide, we know little about the organization of public health infrastructure and health care in world cities. We know even less about the consequences of poor access to health care in these cities, let alone how national health policies influence access to care among city residents. Most studies of urban health focus on poor populations and the organizations and programs that serve them (Gusmano and Rodwin, 2005). These studies are not, however, focused on the city with any intent to improve understanding about how the organization of health services is tied to intrinsic characteristics of cities.

There are some notable exceptions to this pattern. For example, Andrulis and Goodman (1999) published an impressive compendium on the 100 largest cities in the United States with some indicators on the extent of the social safety net. Although one may wonder what the five largest cities in this group have in common with those in the bottom quartile, this dataset is noteworthy because it distinguishes suburbs from central cities and documents important dimensions of the urban health penalty. Andrulis (1997) and colleagues focused primarily on measures of health, including infant mortality and life expectancy. They also compiled data on the use of prenatal care and hospital utilization in these cities. There are, however, few studies on urban (inner city as well as suburban) health system characteristics and outcomes across an international sample of cities. This book helps to address this gap, at least with respect to world cities.

Our comparison of health care in world cities reminds us that there are alternatives to what we find in New York City. Neither the triumphs nor the failures of New York's health care system and of the broader federal and state policies of the United States are inevitable (Klein, 1997; Marmor, Freeman, and Okma, 2005). Examining other systems provides the "gift of perspective" and helps us to understand our own system "by reference to what it is like or unlike" (Marmor, Freeman, and Okma, 2005). As Rudolf Klein explains, "Policy learning . . . is as much a process of self-examination—of reflecting on the characteristics of one's own country and health care system—as of looking at the experience of others . . . the experience of other countries is largely valuable insofar as it prompts a process of critical introspection by enlarging our sense of what is possible and adding to our repertoire of possible policy tools. For policy learning is not about the *transfer* of ideas or techniques . . . but about their adaptation to local circumstances" (Klein, 1997: 1270; emphasis in the original). Indeed, comparative analysis expands our vision of what is possible. Our goal in this book is to stimulate reflection on the consequences of poor access to health care in New York, Paris, and London, and the impact of national health policy for these cities.

When scholars compare cities in the United States with those in other wealthy nations, it is clear that many common "urban problems"—the geographic concentration of poverty, inequality, and poor health—are not distinctive attributes of modern cities. Dreier and colleagues (2004) argue that "cities in Canada, Western Europe, and Australia do not have nearly the same levels of poverty, slums, economic segregation, city-suburb disparities, or even suburban sprawl as does the United States. The question is not whether we can ever solve urban problems but whether we can develop the political will to adopt solutions that can work." Our comparison of health systems across three world cities and their nations generates comparable insights.

Health Systems and Population Health Outcomes: City Comparisons

Increasing urbanization has led to greater awareness that the city is a strategic unit of analysis for understanding the health sector (Vlahov and Gallea, 2002). Yet most health services research—both in the United States and among international organizations such as the World Health Organization (WHO) or the OECD—assumes that nations are the most relevant units of analysis for assessing the performance of health systems and health policy.

Even in the most centralized nations, many challenging problems of health and social policy are passed down to subnational levels. For example, care for vulnerable older persons, people with severe mental illness, the most economically disadvantaged, and the uninsured becomes a kind of residual "hot potato" that is passed on to local governments;

among these, cities bear a disproportionate share of the burden for such health care (Rodwin and Gusmano, 2006a).

Ann and Scott Greer (1983) observed more than two decades ago: "What is striking to those who have been immersed in urban studies and then have become interested in the social response to health and ill health is the extreme segregation of the two areas of inquiry." From the heyday of nineteenth-century European public health movements, which focused on the importance of sanitation (clean water supply, sewers, and garbage disposal) and improvements in housing conditions, to twentieth-century interventions aimed at improving access to health services, the main body of research on public health, as well as on medical care, largely focused on cities. Moreover, the triumph of public health is largely responsible for making cities more habitable. Yet, the field of urban studies has largely ignored the issues of public health and health care (Coburn, 2004). Studies of health care systems have followed the growth of the welfare state in veering away from local territorial concerns and focusing largely on statistical aggregates ranging from regions, states, and nations.

Urban planners typically study cities from perspectives that span architecture, urban design, transportation, economic development, the environment, sociology, anthropology, management, and ecology. Even in great syntheses on the state of cities—for example, Lewis Mumford's *Culture of Cities* (1938), Jane Jacobs's *Death and Life of Great American Cities* (1961), or, more recently, Peter Hall's *Cities in Civilization* (1998)—there is virtually no discussion of the health systems that serve their populations. Likewise, in the official annual reviews by the U.S. Department of Housing and Urban Development on the state of cities (HUD, 1999), there are no chapters on the state of local public health infrastructure or even safety-net services for the uninsured, most of which are left to city and county governments.

In the literature on public health, there are, of course, some classic case studies on the evolution of public health and hospitals in specific cities—for example, Bridgman's *L'Hôpital et la Cité* (1962), Duffy's *History of Public Health in New York City* (1974), Koeppel's *Water for Gotham: A History* (2000), Rivett's *Development of the London Hospital System, 1823–1982* (1986), or Rosner's history of New York's hospitals, *A Once Charitable Enterprise: Hospitals and Health Care in Brooklyn and New York, 1885–1915* (1982). In the broader field of health services research, however, when the city appears as a unit of analysis, it is usually because the investigators either (1) are focused on "inner city" (translation: "poor" and "poor minority") populations that happen to be concentrated in specific inner-city neighborhoods ("concentrated deprivation"); or (2) have selected, unwittingly, a spatial unit that happens to be a neighborhood, a city, or part of a greater metropolitan region. In both cases, however, the choice was driven more by the availability of data or other criteria than by theoretical or practical considerations about how characteristics of cities are related to different aspects of health care systems.

Since the 1970s, a number of studies have begun to address this gap in knowledge. In the United States, Ginzberg, Berliner, and Ostow (1993) compared health care in New York City, Chicago, Los Angeles, and Houston. The International Hospital Federation sponsored a comparative international study, *Health Care in Big Cities* (Paine, 1978). More recently, WHO's Healthy Cities Project led a movement to promote population health in cities throughout the world (Aicher, 1998). Although this project aimed largely at sensitizing local authorities to the health implications of different urban policies, current efforts to evaluate diverse city programs may result in valuable data on the social and economic determinants of health, as well as the role of health systems in affecting population health.

In Europe, the Mégapoles Project (Bardsley, 1999) represents an innovative attempt to combine research and practice by assembling a database on the major capital cities of Europe, their health systems, and the health status of their populations. Along with the compilation of comparative data across these cities, the project has initiated study groups of health and social service professionals to search for relevant innovations in the areas of services for older persons and youth. Although this project is the best-developed attempt to compare population health and health care among cities, it is limited in that the choice of cities was driven by political criteria. Many European capitals (e.g., Vienna and Oslo) are so much smaller than London that one wonders whether cities of such disparate size can learn from one another.

John Wennberg's pioneering research on small-area variations in health care delivery, and the subsequent studies that it spawned, compare the performance of health care systems across small geographic areas, including cities (Wennberg and Gittlesohn, 1973; Wennberg, Freeman, and Culp, 1987). These studies document extensive variations in rates of hospital admission for certain conditions and in rates of surgical procedures between areas that have similar demographic characteristics and similar mortality rates (Perrin et al., 1990). The findings raise important questions about standards of clinical decision-making and the influence of practice styles, reimbursement incentives, and supplier-induced demand.

In contrast to many comparisons of urban health care, much of the literature on small-area variations in health care documents the performance of a local health care system for the entire population, not just the components of the system that address the needs of poor people. The most noteworthy examples of this approach, applied to whole cities, are the comparative analyses of Boston and New Haven (Wennberg, Freeman, and Culp, 1987), which suggest that significant differences in population-based patterns of hospital discharges in these cities do not reflect differences in population health, as measured by mortality. Such findings are critical to the development of further research on the relationship between city characteristics and their health systems.

Our comparison of world cities represents a new approach to the comparison of health systems and cities because it explicitly seeks to compare the health systems and health status among the urban cores of three of the largest cities in OECD nations: New York, Paris, and London.* We demonstrate how a comparison of cities structured around comparable units of analysis provides insights into the interdependence of national and local policy. A number of prominent scholars suggest that the social and economic characteristics of world cities are converging (Friedmann, 1986; Mollenkopf and Castells, 1991; Sassen, 2001).

Peterson (1981) argues that the mobility of capital makes it difficult for these cities to address the social and economic polarization associated with world cities for fear of driving out business. The forces of globalization exacerbate the so-called privileged position of business in capitalist democracies (Dahl, 1985; Elkin 1987; Lindblom, 1977). Because domestic capital has more "exit options" as a result of globalized production, there is at least the perceived or credible risk of domestic capital flight if

---

* The research reported in this book is part of a broader World Cities Project (WCP), which includes Hong Kong and Tokyo as well. We excluded Hong Kong and Tokyo from the analysis of access to health care presented in this book because we have not yet obtained comparable data. For more information about the WCP, see the project website, www.ilcusa.org/pages/projects/world-cities-project.php.

domestic tax and expenditure policies do not favor short-term profitability. Critics assert that the so-called convergence hypothesis advanced by much of the global cities literature underestimates the power of the state and fails to account for important differences in social welfare programs (Body-Gendrot, 1996; Gurr and King, 1987; Savitch and Kantor, 2002; Stone, 1989; White, 1998). This book contributes to the debate by documenting the consequences of national health care policies for residents of three world cities.

For example, even though New York City has one of the largest and most innovative departments of health as well as the largest municipal hospital system in the United States, residents of New York are more likely to die prematurely from conditions amenable to health care and face far more significant financial barriers to primary care than their counterparts in Paris and London. This is particularly true for the city's poorest residents. Indeed, there is greater inequality in access to both primary and specialty health care services among residents of New York City than among residents of either Paris or London. These findings suggest that the "economic determinist" model that dominates the literature on world cities is, at best, incomplete because it fails to account for the national and institutional context within which these cities must operate. The logic of global economic competition may have a profound influence on certain aspects of city life, but national health care systems can either mitigate or exacerbate the often harsh effects of globalization on citizens of world cities.

Although our findings underscore the importance of politics and policy for understanding access to health care in cities, they also highlight the extent to which cities are constrained in their capacity to address the health care needs of their citizens. In the United States, debates about national health care reform should be informed by information about the consequences of poor access to health care in our cities. National policy in the United States has ignored cities for decades; our findings demonstrate the devastating effects of such not-so-benign neglect.

Studies on the Performance of Health Care Systems

To compare these three city health systems and describe the impact of national health policies on them, we must first identify relevant indicators of health system performance. The most difficult issues in evaluating health system performance involve specifying the relationship between the elements of a health care system (inputs and outputs) and their impact on health status (outcomes). But how does one distinguish the effect of health services on health from the effects of improvements in social services, income security, education, and transportation, not to mention individual behaviors as well as the social and physical environment? This question raises the problem of devising indicators of health system performance. It also explains why, in his comparative study of the United States, Sweden, and England, Odin Anderson (1972) found it impossible to attribute differences in the usual health indices of morbidity and mortality to patterns of health care organization in these countries.

Unfortunately, efforts to compare health and social welfare systems in the United States with those of Europe typically have descriptive errors and often address the wrong questions (Gusmano et al., 2007). Comparisons of welfare state spending in the developed world, for example, usually focus on the notion that the United States is a welfare "laggard" (Flora and Heidenheimer, 1981; Wilensky, 1975). Yet, once one broadens the analytic telescope to include indirect as well as direct forms of social welfare, Christopher Howard (1993) argues, effectively, the U.S. "hidden welfare state" is no laggard. Instead of asking why the United States relies on indirect, versus direct, social welfare spending, too many studies focus on why its share of public expenditure is lower. This misleading impression of the U.S. welfare state is problematic because it is impossible to explain welfare policy differences, or to identify policy lessons from the experiences of other nations, if we cannot describe accurately their policies and programs. Marmor and colleagues (2005: 341) argue that "learning about the experiences of other nations is a precondition for understanding why change takes place, or for learning from that experience." Too often, however, comparative studies of the welfare state fail to provide sufficient information about the experiences of other nations.

Likewise, the literature on cross-national comparisons of health care systems often lacks attention to detail and inaccurately describes health care systems abroad. Most studies rely on crude aggregates based on data assembled by organizations such as OECD and WHO (Anderson and Hussey, 2001; Reinhardt, Hussey, and Anderson, 1999; World Bank, 1993; WHO, 2000).

Studies that address health system performance examine a variety of different dimensions and offer a range of criteria for evaluation. One important dimension—public satisfaction—can be traced to the public opinion surveys designed by Robert Blendon, the Gallup Group, Harris Interactive, and Eurobarometer. Whatever the dimensions examined—be they public satisfaction, health outcomes, equity of financing, or a slew of process indicators—the strength of these studies has been to focus attention on differences among health system performance which have, in turn, stimulated the design of more surveys of health systems. The danger in focusing on performance, however, is the temptation to develop a composite indicator for purposes of ranking health care systems. This has encouraged lavish attention from the media on the search for the best health care system, which has become the holy grail of comparative health system performance studies. What is missing in this approach is any effort to understand, assess, and compare health systems in relation to the cultural context, values, and institutions within which "performance indicators" are embedded.

THE WORLD HEALTH ORGANIZATION'S HEALTH SYSTEM PERFORMANCE STUDY

The World Health Organization's 2000 study of health system performance is the most prominent example of the performance-based approach to the comparative analysis of health systems. It ranked the health systems of 191 member states based on "disability-adjusted life expectancy" (DALE), its measure of a nation's health status—and an index based on measures of five objectives: maximizing population health; reducing inequalities in population health; maximizing health system responsiveness; reducing inequalities in responsiveness; and financing health care equitably (WHO, 2000).

Although controversial, the WHO report succeeded in generating tremendous discussion among policy makers and academics about the performance of health systems and the criteria that should be used for evaluating them. Some of the controversy generated by the report can be attributed to complaints from countries that were unhappy about their ranking (Marmor, Freeman, and Okma, 2005), but prominent academics were also critical of the reliance on incomplete and inadequate data, as well as use of questionable methods (Coyne and Hilsenrath, 2002; Marmor, Freeman, and Okma, 2005; Navarro, 2002; Williams, 2001). As one commentary in the *American Journal of Public Health* put it, the data from which the WHO rankings were derived were scant and, in many cases, "missing altogether" (Williams, 2001).

The study's primary indicator of health status, DALE, was constructed from data on the level of disability associated with particular diseases for only 20 of the 191 countries included in the study—and there was no information about the distribution of DALE within each country. Instead, the distribution of childhood mortality, which had to be imputed for most countries, was used as a proxy for the distribution of population health (Reidpath et al., 2003; Richardson, Wildman, and Robertson, 2003; Williams, 2001).

Beyond the issue of missing data and questionable extrapolations, DALE does not differentiate the impact of disability by taking into account the use of compensatory resources (through public and family provision) whose absence transforms a disability into a handicap (Reidpath et al., 2003; Richardson, Wildman, and Robertson, 2003; Rock, 2000). Thus, DALE assumes that the welfare loss experienced by a poor person with a disability in a developing nation that offers little or no access to compensatory technology is comparable to the welfare loss experienced by a wealthy person living in a developed nation with the same disability, even though the latter may live in an environment modified to assist the disabled (Reidpath et al., 2003; Richardson, Wildman, and Robertson, 2003). The WHO's use of DALE also highlights the problem of using broad measures of health status to comment on the performance of health care systems. DALE includes causes of mortality that are amenable to medical care and those that are not. As a result, this measure is not "related directly to the health care system" (Nolte and McKee, 2003: 1129). When Nolte and McKee substituted mortality amenable to health care (a concept that we explore further below and in Chap. 3) for DALE, they found that the country rankings changed substantially. In their analysis, the rankings for many southern European countries, the United Kingdom, and Japan fell, while those for Finland, Norway, Sweden, and New Zealand rose significantly. For an improved understanding of the performance of health care systems and the relationship between health care inputs and health outputs, it is important to select indicators that are more directly related to these systems than such broad measures of population health as life expectancy, potential years of life lost, or DALEs.

The WHO measures of health system "responsiveness" were based on responses to survey questions from a 1,791-person convenience sample. The survey asked respondents to rank their own health systems on a score of 1 (poorest) to 10 (best) on several dimensions of responsiveness.* To capture the distribution of responsiveness within each country, the respondents were also asked to identify groups within their countries that suffered discrimination in this regard. The WHO then calculated "the extent of differences in responsiveness by the subgroups selected by the country's key informants" (Williams, 2001). It also used "as partial evidence the opinions of WHO personnel to 'verify'" claims about each nation (Marmor, Freeman, and Okma, 2005: 345).

The WHO measure of "fair financing" had similar limitations. Using survey data on the percentage of nonfood expenditure spent on health care for 21 countries, the WHO study extrapolated estimates for the other 170 nations. Because this measure of spending on health care was not placed in the context of a country's overall tax burden, it "does not discriminate between systems that are regressive and progressive or between horizontal inequity and progressivity/regressivity" (Richardson, Wildman, and Robertson, 2003: 358).

Beyond these data limitations, efforts to rank health systems are still problematic. The WHO report imposed a universal set of criteria for evaluating health systems. Even if all countries agreed on the broad objectives of health systems, it seems unlikely that they would weight these objectives in the same way. Decisions about the objectives of a country's health system—and the possible tradeoffs that might have to be made among them—are, and should be, political decisions for which "technocratic" solutions are not a substitute (Morone, 1993).

As the discussion of "fair financing" suggests, ranking health system performance can be misleading because such evaluations often take place in a policy vacuum. A country may decide to limit or increase spending on health care services as part of a tradeoff resulting in more or less spending

* These included observation of basic human rights; privacy of consultation and records; choice of treatment options; accessibility and waiting times; cleanliness, food quality, and other amenities; support from community and care agencies; and choice among providers at each level.

on some other good. Alternatively, a country may decide to increase progressivity of health care financing as part of a tradeoff to decrease progressivity in social security financing and social care. Because it is not feasible to incorporate these sorts of tradeoffs into a comparative analysis of health systems, we should exercise great caution before declaring that one system is "better" than another.

THE COMMONWEALTH FUND'S STUDIES OF HEALTH SYSTEM PERFORMANCE

The extensive criticism of the WHO's effort to evaluate health system performance has not discouraged other groups from evaluating health system performance. Most recently, the Commonwealth Fund launched a project designed to identify "high-performing" health systems. Unlike the WHO report, the Commonwealth Fund's project is limited to comparisons between the United States and other wealthy nations. It also draws on significantly more dependable data for its assessments, in part because its scope is more limited and is focused on nations for which population health and health system data are more readily available. For example, it supplements many of the same data sources used by the WHO—including the European Union EuroBarometer Survey of 15 EU countries, the OECD health database, and the WHO mortality database (Davis, 2007)—with original surveys of patients and primary care providers, designed and fielded by Harris Interactive, in Australia, Canada, Germany, New Zealand, the Netherlands, the United Kingdom, the United States, and, more recently, France. Using common sets of questions has enabled the Commonwealth Fund to explore similarities and differences regarding self-reported access to care, the existence and use of clinical information systems, payment incentives, and the use of disease management by primary care physicians in these seven countries (Schoen, Osborn, et al., 2006).

The Commonwealth Fund relies on these survey results, along with a host of other data sources, to compare U.S. national averages on health outcomes, quality, access, efficiency, and equity with "benchmarks," which represent the performance on these measures "achieved by top-performing groups" (Schoen, Davis, et al., 2006). In some cases, the "top-performing groups" are other countries. In other cases, they are regions, states, or health plans within the United States. Despite the more reliable empirical analysis presented by the Commonwealth Fund, its application of benchmarking techniques, and its use of a single national "scorecard" to evaluate the performance of the U.S. health system, such an approach shares many of the same problems of the effort to rank health systems on the basis of criteria promulgated by the WHO.

The benchmarking efforts also raise questions about the appropriate units of comparison. In contrast to theoretical standards, benchmarks based on real-world performance—by other countries, regions, states, or, in some cases, individual health plans operating within the United States— are supposed to provide more "realistic" goals for the nation. Yet, noting that the U.S. average on a host of performance indicators is lower than highest-performing states or plans within the United States is of limited value because this claim is true by definition!

OTHER APPROACHES TO HEALTH SYSTEM PERFORMANCE

Despite the problems of studies on the performance of health systems, there has been progress during the past three decades. Efforts to link health systems characteristics to health outcomes fall into at least four categories: (1) the inventory approach; (2) the production function approach; (3) the avoidable mortality approach (Lefèvre et al., 2004; Nolte and McKee, 2003); and (4) the disease-specific approach (Buck, Eastwood, and Smith, 1999).

The inventory approach focuses on individual health services and attempts to assess the impact of these services on the population at risk by quantifying changes in the associated burden of disease. For example, Bunker and colleagues examined the impact of 13 (clinical) preventive services such as cervical cancer screening and 13 curative services (e.g., treatment of cervical cancer). They estimated that the life-expectancy gain for preventive services is 1.5 years, while the gain for curative services was 3.5–4 years. Taken together, the preventive and curative medical services they examined resulted in about 5 years of a total gain in life expectancy of 30 years (or 17%) during the twentieth century that may be attributed to clinical prevention and curative services (Bunker, Frazier, and Mosteller, 1994).

Some of the initial "inventory" studies were limited because they tried to extrapolate the gains identified in clinical trials to entire populations (Gusmano et al., 2007). More recent studies in this category, however, have employed epidemiological modeling with comparable results. For example, several studies have found that medical and surgical care have produced decreases in mortality due to coronary heart disease (CHD). For England, 42 percent of the decrease in CHD mortality between 1981 and 2000 was attributed to medical and surgical treatments (Unal, Critchley, and Capewell 2004). In Scotland, 44 percent of the fall in CHD mortality between 1975 and 1994 was attributed to these treatments (Capewell, Morrison, and McMurrey, 1999), and in the Netherlands, 46 percent of the decline in CHD mortality was due to treatment (Bots and Grobbee, 1996).

The production function approach analyzes gains in health (the dependent variable)—usually at the national level—as a function of independent variables (Buck, Eastwood, and Smith, 1999), including health care. At the most aggregate level, studies have examined the relationship between health expenditures and health outcomes (Babazono and Hillman, 1994). Frequently, these studies conclude that socioeconomic factors are more important than health care spending (Babazono and Hillman, 1994), but Cremieux and colleagues (1999) showed that within Canada lower health care spending was associated with an increase in infant mortality and a decline in life expectancy, and that this relationship was independent of a number of socioeconomic and lifestyle variables. More specifically, they estimated that a 10 percent reduction in health care spending was associated with higher infant mortality of about 0.5 percent and lower life expectancy of 6 months in men and 3 months in women. A recent cross-country analysis that examined the determinants of health outcomes in 21 OECD countries identified a significant negative relationship between health expenditure and premature mortality among women as measured in potential years of life lost (Or, 2000). A related analysis that assessed the relative importance of medical and nonmedical factors to the decline in premature mortality in OECD countries between 1970 and 1992 showed that more than 60 percent of declines in avoidable mortality among men and 50 percent of declines among women could be attributed to rising health care expenditures.

A subsequent analysis by Or broadened the spectrum of health outcome indicators and took account of nonmonetary health care input variables—for example, number of doctors per capita, as well as type of reimbursement (salary, fee-for-service, capitation) and a measure of access to services (Or, 2001). It showed a strong negative and statistically significant association between the number of doctors and premature mortality, infant mortality, and life expectancy at age 65. Another recent analysis of life expectancy and infant mortality found that increases in health care expenditures are significantly associated with large decreases in infant mortality but only marginally related to life expectancy (Nixon and Ulmann, 2006).

While these studies provide some evidence that the role of health care in the production of population health may be greater than previously assumed, they are limited because the potential and varying time lags between intervention and outcome, which most such regression analyses do not explore in detail (Gravelle and Backhouse, 1987), coupled with the use of cross-sectional data, make it difficult to assess causality.

The avoidable mortality approach focuses on premature deaths due to causes for which the clinical literature suggests there are effective health care interventions that can prevent death before the age of 75 (Charlton et al., 1986; Holland, 1997; Jougla et al., 1987; Lefèvre et al., 2004; Mackenbach et al., 1988; Nolte and McKee, 2003; Poikolainen and Eskola, 1986; Rutstein et al., 1976). The application of this concept to Europe by Nolte and McKee shows that deaths that could have been prevented by timely and effective health care were still relatively common in many countries in 1980. Reductions in these deaths contributed substantially to the overall reduction of premature mortality during the 1980s. The largest contribution was from declining infant mortality rates, but in some countries—including Denmark, France (for men), the Netherlands, Sweden (for women), and the United Kingdom—reductions in deaths among the middle-aged were equally or even more important. In contrast, during the 1990s, reductions in avoidable mortality made a somewhat smaller contribution to reductions in premature mortality, especially in the northern European countries. However, they remained important in southern Europe, especially in Portugal and Greece, where initial death rates had been higher.

The Nolte and McKee findings support the idea that improvements in access to effective health care had a measurable impact in many countries during the 1980s and 1990s, reducing infant mortality and deaths among middle-aged and older persons, particularly women. However, the magnitude of impact has, to a considerable extent, reflected the starting point.

Thus, those countries where infant mortality was relatively high at the beginning of the 1980s, such as Greece and Portugal, saw the greatest reductions in avoidable mortality in infancy. In contrast, in countries where infant mortality rates had already reached very low levels by the beginning of the 1990s, such as Sweden, the scope for further improvement was small.

In a subset of OECD nations, significant work has focused on specific diseases, drawing on individual-level data related to these health conditions. For example, the McKinsey Healthcare Productivity Project compared the management of diabetes mellitus, cholelithiasis (gall stones), lung cancer, and breast cancer in Germany, the United Kingdom, and the United States (Baily and Garber, 1997; McKinsey Global Institute, 1996). The OECD itself has launched the Aging-Related Diseases Project, in which an impressive team of economists has attempted to link treatments with outcomes by collecting comparative data on ischemic heart disease, stroke, and breast cancer (Cutler, 2003; Moise and Jacobzone, 2003).

These studies have yet to yield valid population-based findings across OECD nations, but they have great promise. Other studies with a similar approach are in progress as well. The Commonwealth Fund's International Working Group on Quality Indicators collected data for 21 indicators in Australia, Canada, New Zealand, England, and the United States (Hussey et al., 2004). Their indicators included various dimensions of medical care, including 5-year cancer relative survival rates, 30-day case-fatality rates after acute myocardial infarction and stroke, breast cancer screening, and asthma mortality rates. In her commentary on this study, McGlynn (2004) concluded that there is no perfect health system because each country has at least one area of care in which it excels.

Indicators of Health System Performance for This Study

Our review of attempts to assess the contribution of health care to population health status makes it clear that, to understand the performance of health care systems, we must agree on consistent definitions of health system inputs and population health status. Although financing, cost, and quality are important dimensions of health systems, we focus here on access to timely and effective health services. We have two reasons for limiting our inquiry in this way. First, despite differences in political culture among New York City, Paris, and London, there is broad support for the notion that people who need health care should receive it. Second, there exist comparable measures, at the neighborhood level, in each city, which allow us to evaluate access to health care within and among these cities. The first and broadest measure of access to health care is avoidable mortality. The second measure, more focused on access to primary care, is avoidable hospitalization. The third measure focuses on access to revascularization. These measures allow us to apply our new approach to comparing health system performance among world cities.

We begin by providing a context for comparing access to health care in our three world cities (Chapter 2). In Chapter 3, we explain the logic of avoidable mortality (AM) as an overall measure of health care access. Avoidable mortality does not assume that health care can prevent the occurrence of diseases amenable to screening and medical intervention, but rather, that it should be able to prevent premature death attributed to diseases for which there are effective medical interventions. Among adults, these causes of death include tuberculosis, appendicitis, influenza, pneumonia, ischemic heart disease, and certain forms of cancer. We find that France and Paris have the lowest rates of AM among the three countries and cities we examine, while England and Inner London have the highest rates. Only in Manhattan, however, do residents of the lowest-income neighborhoods have significantly higher rates of AM than the rest of the city.

In Chapter 4, we explain the logic of avoidable hospital conditions (AHCs) as a measure of access to primary care. In discussions about how health systems can assure access through a combination of health insurance coverage, availability of primary care practitioners, and safety net providers, studies in the United States, Canada, Spain, and Britain have recognized AHC as a valid indicator of access to primary care (Brown, Goldacre, and Hicks, 2001; Casanova and Starfield, 1995; Sanderson and Dixon, 2000). AHCs are diagnoses for which access to timely and appropriate primary care services—most significantly, the management of chronic disease—should decrease or avoid the need for hospital admission. Examples of such diagnoses include congestive heart failure, asthma, diabetes, and pneumonia. High rates of hospital admission for AHCs among residents of an area often reflect barriers to primary care and may therefore serve as indicators of access to care (Pappas et al., 1997). Previous research suggests that individuals without health insurance are more likely to be admitted to hospitals with AHCs because they are less likely to receive appropriate and timely ambulatory care than those with insurance (Billings, Anderson, and Newman, 1996; Hadley, Steinberg, and Feder, 1991; Weissman, Gatsonis, and Epstein, 1992). We compare rates of AHCs across and within New York, London, and Paris and investigate factors associated with hospital discharges for AHCs such as age, gender, race, ethnicity, neighborhood-level socioeconomic status, and the number of co-morbid conditions. Although residents of the most deprived boroughs of Inner London experience higher rates of AHCs than do residents in the least deprived boroughs, we find the greatest disparities in rates of AHCs within Manhattan. African-Americans, Hispanics, residents without private health insurance, and residents of Manhattan's lowest-income neighborhoods are hospitalized with avoidable conditions at a particularly high rate.

Finally, in Chapter 5, we investigate the availability and use of specialty care by focusing on the treatment of heart disease. Despite a recent decline in deaths from ischemic heart disease (IHD), this disease remains the world's leading cause of death, as well as a major contributor to health care expenditures. Cross-national comparisons that assess dimensions of health system performance indicate that the United States has higher rates of cardiac catheterization and revascularization procedures—percutaneous transluminal coronary angioplasty (PTCA) and coronary artery bypass graft (CABG) surgery—than France, the United Kingdom, and other wealthy nations (OECD, 2000). A study based on the most recent state-of-the-art international comparison on the use of high-tech interventions concludes that the United States is more aggressive than Canada, Scotland, Sweden, Israel, Australia, and Denmark in providing revascularization procedures following heart attacks (Technological Change in Health Care Research Network, 2001).

Yet, few comparative studies attempt to account for differences in the burden of heart disease when comparing rates of revascularization. To assess the relationship between treatment rates and the prevalence of IHD we present a simple index based on the ratio of procedure rates to hospital discharge rates for acute myocardial infarction (AMI). We find that once we account for differences in disease across these countries and cities, the United States appears to be less of an outlier. This pattern is even more striking when we focus on the cities that have more comparable health care delivery systems. The comparison between Manhattan and Paris, in particular, is remarkable. When we account for differences in heart disease across the urban cores of these cities, we find that Parisians receive more revascularizations at every age group than do residents of Manhattan, and residents of France age 65 years and older receive more of these procedures than do their counterparts in the United States.

We are also able to highlight similar gender disparities in the treatment of heart disease. Heart disease is usually considered a "man's disease" because the rate of heart disease is much higher among men than women, particularly before the age of 65, yet heart disease is the leading cause of death among women. Moreover, recent clinical studies indicate that women are systematically underdiagnosed and undertreated. Despite these findings, advocates for women's health have, until recently, focused on other health issues. We examine gender differences within and among our selected countries and cities while adjusting for the prevalence of disease. We find that among persons diagnosed with heart disease, women are significantly less likely to receive a revascularization, after controlling for age and, to the extent possible, morbidity.

Summary

There are few comparative studies of New York, Paris, and London—and fewer still that examine their health care systems and population health. Because these three world cities have a great deal in common, comparisons of their health care systems provide insights into the possible effects of national and local policies on the use of health services and population health status. In addition, the experience of these three cities in establishing public health infrastructure, developing health care systems, and attempting to overcome their own inequalities among diverse neighborhoods may provide useful lessons in meeting the daunting challenges of megacities in developing nations.

Despite the growth of urbanization worldwide, we know surprisingly little about the consequences of poor access to health care in world cities, let alone how national health policies influence access to care among city residents. This book helps to fill this gap in knowledge. Our aim is to stimulate policy makers in each city and its respective nation to reflect not only on the consequences of poor access to health care in New York, Paris, and London, but also on the impact of national health policy for cities.

CHAPTER TWO

Comparable Cities within Contrasting Health Systems

I N THIS CHAPTER we provide a context for comparing access to health care in New York City, Paris, and London. We review the evolution of health systems in wealthy nations and compare their salient features in the United States, France, and England. We then describe the defining characteristics of the health care systems and public health infrastructure in these three cities. Finally, we develop our rationale and framework for comparing these cities. We identify the relevant geographic boundaries, review the similarities and differences across these cities, and compare the size and structure of their health services systems.

The Evolution of National Health Care Systems

Although leaders in New York City, Paris, and London imagine their world cities to be unique places, their health care systems and public health infrastructure, while being embedded within distinct national health systems, all nevertheless evolved in similar directions over the twentieth century. The essential point of convergence across these systems is that national governments have gradually extended their role in the financing and organization of health care services. What was once largely the responsibility of the family, philanthropy, religious institutions, and local governments has largely been taken over by national and subnational governments—a trend that has accompanied the rise of the welfare state (De Kervasdoué, Kimberly, and Rodwin, 1984). This evolution has affected all wealthy nations that constitute the majority members of the Organization for Economic Cooperation and Development (OECD).

The pattern of increasing government expenditure and intervention in the health sector became more pronounced in the decades following

World War II, to the point where most people have benefited from many dimensions of this government largesse. Even in the United States, where conservatives have resisted this trend, few could claim not to have benefited—directly or indirectly—from hospitals that were granted tax-exempt status or other government subsidies, health professionals who were trained with government grants, medical research that was financed by the federal government, private health insurance that was tax deductible to an employer, or a host of public health programs, including Medicaid and Medicare.

The growth of government involvement in health care systems characterized OECD nations during the great boom years of health sector growth (the 1950s and 1960s), when governments encouraged hospital construction and modernization, workforce training, and biomedical research. It continued in the 1970s, when the goals shifted more in the direction of rationalization and cost containment (Rodwin, 1984). In the twenty-first century, as public and other forms of collective private financing (e.g., health insurance) have become the dominant sources of funding for health care, public expenditure on health care services has become the largest category of social expenditure, as a share of gross domestic product (GDP), after Social Security payments. Furthermore, in the United States and other countries, governments have increasingly broadened the scope of their intervention to encompass new regulatory functions.

These trends are so powerful that they have affected the way we conceptualize health care systems. Indeed, the comparative study of health systems is dominated by attention to the role of the nation-state. Thus, we move on to provide an overview of contrasting health care systems across OECD nations. Next, we provide more in-depth information about the health systems in the United States, France, and England.

AN OVERVIEW OF CONTRASTING HEALTH CARE SYSTEMS

The U.S. health care system is a complex patchwork of public and private insurance with large gaps in coverage. It is the most expensive health care system in the world, yet more than 47 million people in the United States have no health insurance, and the health status of the population is poor in comparison with that of most other wealthy nations. The English National Health Service is financed largely on the basis of general revenue taxes. It emphasizes free care at the point of delivery and aims to provide care on the basis of patient "need." While pursuing these lofty goals, the NHS is severely constrained by its budget—the lowest among wealthy nations; there are consequently frequent complaints about the degree to which it limits the supply of doctors and hospitals, delays the adoption of new medical technology, and results in waiting lists for its patients. France has a system of national health insurance (NHI), which, after a series of incremental expansions, now covers 99 percent of the population. The French NHI is one of the most expensive systems in Europe, but it is noted for providing extensive access to primary as well as specialty care.

Whether one's image of a health system is private and market-based, as in the United States and Switzerland, or public and state-controlled, as in Great Britain and Scandinavian nations, or at some intermediary point along such a continuum, as in France, Canada, and Japan, it is possible to make some useful distinctions with respect to the financing and organization of health services. The matrix in Table 2.1 can help classify health systems by distinguishing methods of health care financing (columns) and categories of organizational arrangements (rows).

The four sources of funding to pay for health services are the government (general revenue funds through the fiscal tax system); Social Security/national health insurance (funds from compulsory payroll taxes); private insurance (funds raised through voluntary premiums assessed by private

TABLE 2.1.   The financing and organization of health systems: a typology

Organizational arrangement		Financing source		
	(A) Government	(B) Social Security or NHI	(C) Private insurance	(D) Out of pocket
		Type number		
(A) Government owned	1	2	3	4
(B) Private nonprofit/ quasi-government	5	6	7	8
(C) Private for-profit	9	10	11	12

SOURCE: Rodwin, 2006a.

health insurance companies); and out-of-pocket payments from individual patient payments. There are, of course, other minor sources of health care financing, particularly for capital expenditures—for example, direct employer contributions and philanthropic funds. But these are no longer major categories of financing for health care services.

The organizational arrangements in Table 2.1 refer to the supply of health services: public, private not-for-profit, or private for-profit. Within these categories, many distinctions may be added. For example, in the United States, some publicly capitalized organizations (row A) are national (the Veterans Administration), others are subnational (state mental hospitals), and many are local (municipal hospitals). Likewise, the not-for-profit category (row B) may include a variety of quasi-public organizations (e.g., hospital trusts and foundations in Great Britain). The for-profit form of organization (row C), an important subcategory in the United States, would include investor-owned hospitals and managed care organizations (MCOs). Indeed, the growth of large investor-owned MCOs distinguishes the health care system of the United States from that of most other OECD nations. This simple matrix enables one to highlight some classic health system models and to think about the three urban health care systems we examine in this book within this broader cross-national perspective.

NATIONAL HEALTH SERVICE SYSTEMS

National health service systems—such as those in Great Britain, Sweden, Norway, Finland, Denmark, Portugal, Spain, Italy, and Greece—are typically traced back to Lord Beveridge, who wrote the blueprint for the British NHS immediately following World War II. In such systems a dominant share of financing is derived from taxes (column 1 of Table 2.1). Likewise, their systems of hospital provision have been dominated by public sector organizational forms (row A) that are now coming to resemble quasi-public organizations in Great Britain (row B). These general characteristics do not preclude other forms of financing (columns B, C, and D), nor do they preclude a significant mix of other associated organizational forms (rows B and C). Indeed, some of the most interesting differences among NHS systems revolve around the extent to which they combine a different mix of the financing and organizational forms represented by the columns and rows of Table 2.1. For example, the relative proportion of private financing and provision is much higher in Italy and Spain than in Sweden or Denmark. Another distinguishing characteristic of NHS systems is their tendency to rely largely on budgets to allocate government resources in the health sector and control total health care expenditures. National health insurance systems, by contrast, have had a more open-ended reimbursement system for health care providers, although this distinction is rapidly blurring as NHI systems are increasingly under pressure to operate within budget limits.

NATIONAL HEALTH INSURANCE SYSTEMS

National health insurance (NHI) systems like those in France, Austria, Belgium, Luxembourg, and Japan were all influenced by Chancellor Otto von Bismarck's NHI program for salaried industrial workers in Germany in 1883. These systems tend to be characterized by a dominant share of financing from column B. Canada is an exception to this pattern because the dominant share of financing is from general tax revenues. Likewise, NHI systems of provision are characterized by a more balanced public-private mix than in NHS systems. Once again, these general characteristics do not preclude the contributions of other forms of financing (columns A, C, and D). Nor do they preclude a dominance of public hospitals in nations such as France and Germany (row A).

As with NHS systems, NHI systems are also characterized by significant variation in their financing and organizational arrangements. For example, the share of French health care expenditures that is financed from general tax revenues (column A) has increased beyond 40 percent. Likewise, the relative share of proprietary hospital beds ranges widely across NHI systems from none in Canada to 23 percent in France.

AN EMERGING PARADIGM?

A look at Table 2.1 suggests that it is hard to locate any existing health system within any one box. Because of the enormous pluralism of the United States, components of its health system are within every one of these boxes. Among most OECD nations, which include Japan and the United States, no existing systems actually correspond to the pure NHI and NHS models. In fact, most health systems in wealthy nations have converged along the lines of what Hurst has called the "contractual model" (Hurst and Poullier, 1993). This model indicates that there is an important dimension missing in Table 2.1: the relationships between health care purchasers and providers. Chernichovsky (1995, 2002) analyzes this emerging paradigm in relation to what he calls the "organization and management of care consumption" (OMCC).

The contractual model and the functions of OMCC suggest that what is important in the comparative analysis of OECD health systems— beyond the question of how to finance health services or how to achieve the right balance among public and private organizational arrangements— is how to allocate available resources to achieve the best results. This challenge raises issues of health system performance, governance, accountability, consumer control, management of care, and overall integration of health services across the full continuum of care.

Financing Health Care

THE U.S. PATCHWORK OF PUBLIC
AND PRIVATE INSURANCE

The United States relies on a mix of public and private financing with multiple payers. Although the United States has the highest per capita health care expenditures—for public and private combined—among the wealthy OECD nations and spends the highest percentage of its GDP on health care, it retains the lowest share of public expenditure as a percentage of total health expenditures.

Most Americans under the age of 65 with health insurance have employer-sponsored private health insurance. The expansion of employer-paid health insurance during the 1950s and 1960s was induced by a series of administrative, legal, and legislative decisions, none of which was explicitly intended to expand employer involvement in health care. As Christopher Howard (1993) noted, because the United States relies on "tax expenditures" to subsidize private welfare benefits like employer-sponsored health insurance, the true scope of the U.S. welfare state is "hidden."

By the end of the 1950s, employers had a substantial role in the financing of health care, along with a number of other fringe benefits. Approximately three-quarters of the 123 million Americans with private health insurance obtained coverage through the workplace (Field and Shapiro, 1993: 71). Employer-based coverage continued to expand through the 1960s, stabilizing in the early 1970s. Since 2000, the percentage of employers who offer health insurance coverage has declined, along with the percentage of employees who take up the offer of employer-sponsored health insurance. Although a small portion of this decline may be due to the expansion of public health insurance coverage, particularly the State Child Health Insurance Program (SCHIP), most of the decline in employer offers and employee take-up is due to increases in health insurance premiums (Reschovsky et al., 2006). In addition to this decline among current workers, many employers have reduced or eliminated retiree health benefits (Gottschalk, 2007). It is not clear whether these reductions represent the end of employer-based health insurance, as some suggest, but no one disputes that it has eroded substantially (Gottschalk, 2007).

Although coverage through the development of a private, employment-based health insurance system expanded over the 1950s and 1960s, many Americans were left behind. Most obviously, this publicly subsidized private system did not address the health needs of those who were not in the workforce, particularly the unemployed and older persons (Starr, 1982: 333). The adoption of Medicare and Medicaid in 1965 attempted to fill these gaps. After a nearly 15-year struggle that began during the Truman administration, Medicare was passed in 1965, along with a "welfare bill" to be administered by the states known as Medicaid (Marmor, 1973).

The Social Security Amendments of 1965 (the Medicare and Medicaid legislation) included three distinct layers. The first layer was Medicare Part A. Based on President Johnson's original proposal, Part A is a hospital insurance program based on the Social Security contributory model. The second layer was Medicare Part B. Part B was based on a proposal from Republican Congressman John Byrnes of Ohio and is a voluntary supplementary medical insurance program funded through beneficiary premiums and federal general revenues. The third and final layer was the Medicaid program, based on the proposal from the American Medical Association (AMA) and other opponents of the president's hospital social insurance plan. Medicaid broadened the protections offered to the poor under medical vendor payments and to the medically indigent under

Kerr-Mills. The Kerr-Mills means test was also changed to cover additional older citizens, and eligibility among the indigent was broadened to include the blind, the permanently disabled, and adults in (largely) single-headed families and their dependent children (Grogan and Gusmano, 2007).

Despite occasional flirtations with the idea of expanding Medicare and reducing the age of eligibility,* the scope of the Medicare program has not changed radically since its adoption in 1965 (Brown and Sparer, 2003). In 1972, the program was expanded to include the disabled and people with end-stage renal disease, but the most significant change in the program's scope and structure came with the 2003 Medicare Modernization Act. Most of the public attention was devoted to the creation of Medicare "Part D," a new prescription drug benefit. Along with the creation of a prescription drug benefit, the act also provided incentives to encourage beneficiaries to select Medicare Advantage (MA) plans over the traditional Medicare program (Marmor and Mashaw, 2006; White, 2007). By July 2006, about 16 percent (7.3 million) of Medicare beneficiaries were enrolled in Medicare Advantage plans, an increase of 3 percent over the year before (White, 1998).

In contrast to Medicare, which has experienced few increases in scope during its 40-year history, the Medicaid program has grown enormously, particularly since the late 1980s. In the late 1980s a group of southern governors pushed to liberalize coverage for pregnant women under Medicaid. Congress and President George H. W. Bush approved the expansion because they supported the goal of reducing infant mortality through the expanded use of prenatal care and because the expansion was supposed to remain "budget neutral" (Sparer, 2007). By 1990, the federal government had expanded Medicaid to include all pregnant women and children with incomes below 133 percent of the federal poverty level and required states to phase in coverage of all children in families with incomes below 100 percent of poverty (Sparer, 2007). After remaining stable for 20 years, Medicaid enrollment grew from about 20 million in 1986 to about 40 million in 1993 (Sparer, 2007).

* Representative Pete Stark (CA), among others, proposed "Medicare for All," which would allow the Medicare program to serve as a single-payer system for the entire country. During the second Clinton administration there were proposals to extend Medicare eligibility to persons 50 years of age and older.

In 1997, the State Child Health Insurance Program expanded public insurance coverage for children even further. After the failure of the Clinton health plan in 1994, congressional Democrats decided to build on the Medicaid expansions of the late 1980s. Republicans opposed a further expansion of Medicaid but supported a block grant program to expand coverage for working-class children. The two parties reached a compromise, and SCHIP was created as a separate program with a funding model that is similar to Medicaid because it provides federal matching funds for state programs that enjoy significant discretion (Brown and Sparer, 2003). The federal government provided states with $40 billion over 10 years to provide expanded child coverage. As of 2007, SCHIP covered more than 6.1 million children (AcademyHealth, 2007). Soon after taking office, President Obama signed legislation providing an additional $33 billion to SCHIP. This funding is expected to provide insurance to about 4 million children (Levey, 2009).

Despite the patchwork of public and private insurance described above, more than 47 million Americans do not have health insurance. To care for the uninsured, the United Sates relies on a makeshift "system" of safety net providers, including public and not-for-profit hospitals, federally qualified community health centers, school-based health centers, municipal/local health clinics, nonprofit Visiting Nurse Associations, family planning clinics, and public dental clinics. Together, these institutions play a vital role in providing access to the uninsured and Medicaid clients, but the growth in the number of uninsured and reductions in payments from public and private payers has undermined their ability to do so. In 2000, the Institute of Medicine (IOM) concluded that the safety net was "intact but endangered" (Lewin and Altman, 2000).

THE FRENCH NATIONAL HEALTH INSURANCE

The French health care system achieved note after it was ranked number 1 in the World Health Organization's Millennium Report (WHO, 2000). Although the report's methodology has been criticized (Coyne and Hilsenrath, 2002), indicators of health status, access to services, overall satisfaction, and health care expenditures do support the view that France's health care system is impressive. For decades, French politicians have defended their health system as an ideal lying somewhere between Britain's "nationalized" health service, where there is too much rationing, and the U.S. "competitive" health care system, where there are too many people without health insurance.

In stark contrast to the United States, French national health insurance (NHI) covers the entire population legally residing in France who have met the basic residency requirements (Rodwin, 2003). While co-payments result in out-of-pocket expenditures, most of the population has always had complementary insurance through a system that resembles Medigap coverage for U.S. Medicare beneficiaries (Rodwin and LePen, 2005). In contrast to Medicare, French NHI coverage increases when a patient's costs increase; there are no deductibles; and pharmaceutical benefits are extensive. Moreover, patients with debilitating or chronic illness are exempted from paying coinsurance. Out-of-pocket payments as a share of all health care expenditures are among the lowest among OECD nations.

French NHI is financed largely by employer (45%) and employee (13%) payroll taxes and a "general social contribution" (41%) levied by the French treasury on all earnings, including investment income (Commission des Comptes de la Sécurité Sociale, 2002). In terms of payroll tax rates, employers pay 12.8 percent on all wages, and employees pay 0.75 percent. Employees also pay 7.5 percent of their wages toward the general social contribution. In terms of total personal health expenditures, French NHI contributes 79 percent, supplementary private insurance covers 8 percent (5% for the nonprofit sector—*mutuelles*—and 3% for the commercial sector), and out-of-pocket expenditures represent 13 percent.

The broad contours of the present system of NHI in France were implemented following World War II. As in Great Britain, France developed a welfare state, but its institutional form differed from that outlined in the Beveridge Report. In Britain, the state increased its control over the health system through the nationalization of hospitals and the establishment of a national health service. In France, the state increased its control more gradually while involving business groups (the *patronat*) and trade unions in the management of the social security system. As Ashford (1980) observed, Great Britain created its welfare state "by intent" and France "by default." The paradoxical result is that France far outspends Britain in the health and social services sector. The only similarity between these nations is the centralized and powerful role of the state in the management of the health care system.

French NHI evolved in stages from its original passage in 1928, in which only 14 percent of the population was covered, to its implementation of universal coverage in January 2000, which extended comprehensive first-dollar coverage to the remaining 1 percent of the uninsured population (Couverture Maladie Universelle, or CMU). In 1945, NHI was extended to all salaried employees and their dependents with the goal of including the entire population. The process took the rest of the century to complete. In 1961, farmers and agricultural workers were covered, in 1966 independent professionals were brought into the scheme, and in 1974 another law proclaimed that NHI should be universal.

French Social Security is typically depicted, following an agrarian metaphor, as a set of three sprouting branches: (1) pensions—what we call Social Security in the United States; (2) family allowances—our earned income credit, and more; and (3) health insurance and workplace accidents (occupational health) (Dupeyroux, 1996). Since 1967, each branch has been managed by a national fund with the exception of the third branch, which is run by three principal national funds: the NHI Fund for Salaried Workers (Caisse Nationale d'Assurance Maladie des Travailleurs Salariés, CNAMTS); the NHI Fund for Farmers and Agricultural Workers (Mutualité Sociale Agricole, MSA); and the NHI Fund for the Independent Professions (artisans and self-employed professionals) (Caisse Nationale d'Assurance Maladie des Professions Indépendantes, CANAM).

In addition to these principal NHI funds, there are 18 smaller funds for specific occupations and their dependents—government employees, the military, merchant seamen, miners, railway workers, subway workers, notaries public, artists, and others—all of whom defend their "rightfully earned" entitlements under French NHI. Eleven of these funds are administered by the CNAMTS, which covers 84 percent of legal residents in France and CMU beneficiaries. CANAM and MSA cover, respectively, 8 and 6 percent of the population. The others—less than 1 percent of the population—have their own autonomous organizations operating within the prescribed statutory framework.

All of the national funds responsible for managing French NHI are legally private organizations responsible for the provision of a public service. This makes them, in effect, quasi-public organizations supervised by the ministry in charge of French Social Security. The principal NHI funds have a network of local and regional funds under their administrative control. These organizations function somewhat like American fiscal intermediaries in the management of Medicare. They cut reimbursement checks for health care providers, look out for fraud and abuse, and provide a range of customer services for beneficiaries of their funds.

THE ENGLISH NATIONAL HEALTH SERVICE

The English NHS is financed almost entirely through general revenue taxation and is accountable directly to the central government's Department of Health and Social Security (DHSS) and Parliament. Access to health services is free of charge to all British subjects and to all legal residents. Despite such universal entitlement, health expenditures in the United Kingdom represent only 7.7 percent of the GDP—about one-half that in the United States.

In 2000, the British government adopted a plan (U.K. Department of Health, 2000) noted for its resolve that the NHS would cease to be "a 1940s system operating in a 21st century world." In striking contrast to the health expenditures in wealthier OECD nations, which average 10 percent, the NHS plan called for raising the level of expenditures from 6.7 to 8 percent of GDP in 2006—the average level in the European Union (Klein, 2001). This objective was supported by a tax increase in 2003, which was designed to finance NHS spending by an average of 7.4 percent (in real terms) a year for the next 5 years (Stevens, 2004). These expenditure increases have already served to increase medical school intake by 55 percent, and the number of nurses by 50,000 (since 1997), through pay incentives, return-to-work schemes for doctors with young children, and international recruitment (Stevens, 2004). In addition they allowed for the building of new hospitals and the modernization of old ones and a £2.3 billion investment in electronic health records over the next three years. Finally, the new funds are supporting the new NHS Modernization Agency, which aims to improve programs for cancer, cardiac, and primary care, as well as elective surgery.

Beyond new resources, there is a new effort to implement "national service frameworks" and attain detailed targets for health system improvement, including better treatment outcomes along a whole range of specific indicators. To assist in this objective a new infrastructure of inspection and regulation has been established. There will be published information on performance and financial incentives for providers who excel. But perhaps more important of all, the problems of inefficiency, lack of integration, and inadequate responsiveness to consumers have been confronted by devolving 75 percent of NHS funding to some 300 local NHS primary care trusts (PCTs) all of which are capitated payers now responsible for purchasing a continuum of health services for the populations within their geographic areas.

Paying Providers

THE UNITED STATES

Before the spread of managed care in the 1990s, private insurance in the United States relied primarily on retrospective fee-for-service payments to physicians and other health care providers. Public and private payers in the United States now use a variety of reimbursement methods that include fee-for-service payments and capitation. In the public sector, Medicare relies on a type of negotiated fee-schedule called the resource-based relative value scale (RBRVS). The RBRVS payment formula attempts to account for the resource costs needed to provide each physician service. Physicians may choose to sign a participating agreement and accept RBRVS as payment in full. If they choose not to participate, they may bill patients for charges that exceed the RBRVS allowance.* If they choose to be private contracting physicians, they may bill patients directly and forego any payments from Medicare.†

Medicare Advantage plans and most Medicaid MCOs receive capitated payments that cover both ambulatory and hospital care. In both Medicare and Medicaid managed care, MCOs use a host of reimbursement mechanisms to pay the health care providers in their networks.

---

* There are limits on extra billing from nonparticipating physician. These additional charges may not exceed 115% of the Medicare-approved amount for nonparticipating physicians. Effectively, this limits the extra charge to 9.25% of the RBRVS formula for participating physicians because Medicare rates for nonparticipating physicians are 95% of the rates for participating physicians. Some states require physicians to accept Medicare payments as payments in full—and some physicians are required by contracts with hospitals or managed care plans to participate in the Medicare program.

† The "private contracting" option was established in 1997. Once a physician decides to opt out of Medicare, he or she may not submit claims to Medicare for a 2-year period.

The original reimbursement standards used by the Medicare program were generous and paid hospitals and physicians on a retrospective basis (Morone and Dunham, 1985: 274). Under the prospective payment system adopted in 1983, Medicare set standard payments for hospitalization. This system was made possible by the development of a classification scheme consisting of 467 diagnosis-related groups (DRGs). Medicare payments are predetermined on the basis of the patient's diagnosis, after adjusting for the average cost of care for that DRG in the area. Once the hospital determines the diagnosis, Medicare reimburses the hospital on the basis of the set price, regardless of the costs the hospital bears for treating the beneficiary. In theory, this system forces hospitals to become more efficient. If a hospital is able to treat a patient for less than it is reimbursed under the DRG, it is allowed to keep the difference. When it costs more to treat a patient than the DRG rate, the hospital loses money.*

FRANCE

In France, physicians in the ambulatory sector and in private hospitals are reimbursed on the basis of a negotiated fee schedule. Approximately 30 percent of all physicians select the option to extra-bill beyond the negotiated fees that represent payment in full for the remaining 70 percent of physicians, although this varies by specialty and location. They may extra-bill as long as their charges are presented with "tact and measure," a standard that has never been legally defined but which has been found, empirically, to represent a 50 to 100 percent increase to the negotiated fees. Physicians based in public hospitals are reimbursed on a part-time or full-time salaried basis.

Private hospitals used to be reimbursed according to a negotiated per diem fee; in the late 1990s this system gradually changed to a case-mix reimbursement system. Beginning in 1984, public hospitals were reimbursed on the basis of prospectively set "global" budgets adjusted for patient case mix. This system was inspired by the case-based methods (DRGs) developed in the United States. The most recent modification, a prospective

---

* Initially, critics argued that this financial incentive, rather than leading to more "efficient" care, led hospitals to release patients "quicker and sicker" (Litman and Robins 1991).

payment system, was introduced in 2004 (Schreyögg et al., 2006). Since July 2005, France has used the same reimbursement system, although with different tariffs, for public and private hospitals (Schreyögg et al., 2006).

In 1996, as part of a broader reform of the Social Security system, Prime Minister Juppé attempted the most far-reaching reform of the French health sector since 1958 (LePen and Rodwin, 1996). The central state's supervisory role over the NHI system was reinforced. In addition, the French Parliament was made accountable for health expenditures. It was required to set a global target for total health care expenditures reimbursed by the French NHI and to set targets for each of France's 21 regions. To advise Parliament in this new responsibility and assist the Ministry of Health in overseeing the health system, a slew of new institutions were created: the National Committee on Public Health, the National Agency for Hospital Accreditation and Quality, and regional agencies for hospital planning and control.

Although President Chirac dissolved Parliament in 1996 shortly after the national strikes in protest of the Social Security reforms, almost all of the health care reforms were maintained by the socialist government of Prime Minister Jospin (1997–2002). Perhaps most noteworthy has been the increased role of the National Agency on Health Accreditation and Evaluation in setting standards for the quality of hospital care and developing national medical guidelines for physicians in private practice, which the NHI administration is trying to enforce.

ENGLAND

In the NHS, about two-thirds of general practitioners and dentists are private contractors and are reimbursed through a mixed payment system that includes a basic practice allowance, fee-for-service payments for targeted services, and capitation. Capitation now makes up most of the reimbursement to general practitioners (Oliver, 2005).

Primary care trusts are responsible for purchasing hospital and specialty medical care services for their NHS patients. Before 2003, PCTs used nonbinding block contracts, based on historic costs, to purchase these services. The NHS first introduced a prospective payment system for reimbursing public and private hospitals in 2003 and in April 2004 started phasing in a new national tariff system. PCTs continue to negotiate contracts with hospitals and other providers, but prices are set by the Department of Health, using national prospective tariffs for each Health-care Resource Group (HRG). HRGs are based loosely on U.S. DRGs and are supposed to promote choice, efficiency, and quality. By setting the same tariff for inpatient and day cases, for example, HRGs provide a financial incentive for hospitals to care for as many patients as possible on an outpatient basis (Schreyögg et al., 2006).

Delivery Systems: Organization and Capacity

Organizational arrangements for health care in the United States are noted for being on the private end of the public-private spectrum. In comparison with Western Europe, the United States has one of the smallest public hospital sectors. The absence of an NHI program has resulted in a system of multiple public and private health insurers and has encouraged a more pluralistic pattern of health care organization and more innovative forms of medical practice—for example, multispecialty group practices, health maintenance organizations (HMOs), ambulatory surgery centers, preferred provider organizations (PPOs), and "point of service" (POS) plans.

The United States also differs from Canada and Western Europe with regard to the ways in which health resources are used. For example, the United States (along with Spain and the United Kingdom) is among those OECD countries with the lowest number of acute care hospital beds per 1,000 population. These data should not necessarily lead one to the conclusion that the United States is less prone to institutionalize patients than Western Europe and Canada. Instead, they probably reflect the size of the American private nursing home industry, which has no equivalent in Western Europe or Canada, where a portion of long-term care for older persons is still provided in hospitals.

Despite these important differences between the United States and other OECD nations, the image of a mainly private organizational structure in American health care is misleading and incomplete. In spite of a notable but small investor-owned hospital sector, a dominant investor-owned managed care sector, and the relatively small size of the public sector in the United States in comparison with OECD nations, the government nevertheless plays an important role in the U.S. health care system—both in ambulatory services for non-institutionalized patients and in the provision of hospital services. Almost 30 percent of all registered hospitals (private, nonprofit, local, state, and federal) are owned and operated by governments (AHA, 2000). This sector includes federal Veterans Health Administration hospitals, marine and military hospitals, as well as state, county, and municipal hospitals.

Although the French health care system was ranked number 1 on the basis of overall efficiency and fairness by the WHO study of health system performance (WHO, 2000), it still has several problems. From a public health point of view, there is inadequate communication between full-time salaried physicians in public hospitals and solo-based private practice physicians working in the community. Although general practitioners in the fee-for-service sector (who account for roughly one-half of French physicians) have informal referral networks to specialists and public hospitals, there are no formal institutional relationships that assure continuity of medical care, disease prevention and health promotion services, posthospital follow-up care, and more generally, systematic linkages and referral patterns between primary-, secondary-, and tertiary-level services.

Since its creation in 1948, Great Britain's NHS has been one of the largest public service organizations in Europe. With more than a million employees, more than 2,500 hospitals, and a host of intermediary health care organizations, the NHS poses an awesome managerial challenge. NHS resources are extremely scarce by OECD standards. Perhaps because of this and because the NHS faces the same demands as other systems to make available technology and to care for an increasingly aged population, the British have been more aggressive in weeding out inefficiency and pursuing innovations that improve efficiency. But there have been numerous obstacles in the way: opposition by professional bodies, difficulties in firing and redeploying health care personnel, and the tripartite structure of the NHS, which, since its inception, has created an institutional separation between hospitals, general practitioners, and community health programs.

This institutional framework of regional health authorities (RHAs) for hospitals, family practitioner committees (recently greatly empowered and called primary care trusts), and local authorities has created perverse incentives—for example, to shift some patients back and forth from general practitioners to hospital physicians (known as "consultants"), to the community, and back to the hospital. Until the reforms introduced by the Thatcher government in 1991, general practitioners had no incentive to minimize costs and could even impose costs on RHAs by referring patients to hospital consultants or for diagnostic services. NHS managers could shift costs from the NHS to Social Security by sending elderly hospitalized patients to private nursing homes. Hospital consultants could attempt to shift costs back to the patient by keeping long waiting lists, thereby increasing demand for their services paid privately. As in France, neither patients nor physicians in Britain bear the cost of the decisions they make; it is the taxpayer who pays the bill.

In July 1990, RHAs were streamlined, and family practitioner committees were transformed into newly named "family health service authorities" (FHSAs) with stronger management over primary care. In 1996 the districts were merged with the FHSAs into roughly 80 health authorities and placed under a new National Health Service Executive with eight regional offices. The health authorities were supposed to function as integrated purchasing coalitions, thereby strengthening the role of competition and internal markets in the allocation of health resources (Smee, 2000).

Following Tony Blair's election as prime minister in 1997, the New Labour Party's "third way" reforms focused more on collaboration and less on competition, but the government's white paper retained the major elements of the Thatcher reforms (U.K. Department of Health, 1989). The purchaser/provider split was retained, albeit with more emphasis on co-operation. All general practitioners have now been incorporated into PCTs, thus bringing important elements of managed care to the NHS. Fundholders have now been largely absorbed by PCTs, and the health authorities are losing their former purchasing role as they become increasingly responsible for providing a framework for PCT accountability (Dobson, 1999). Finally, as in France and Canada, there have been efforts to improve quality and standards. The National Institute for Health and Clinical Effectiveness is setting standards and the Council for Health Improvement is supposed to enforce them (Le Grand, 1999).

Comparable Cities: An Overview of Health Care Systems and Public Health Infrastructure

New York, Paris, and London have confronted devastating infectious disease epidemics over the past two centuries. In response, to protect their population's health and avert potential catastrophes, these cities have developed a diverse set of institutions reflecting their distinctive institutional and cultural characteristics. Although they all have well-known centers of medical excellence and a concentration of health care resources within their urban cores, they differ with respect to their systems of health care coverage, the organization of their hospitals and primary care systems, and the overall organization of their public health infrastructure. These differences, of course, reflect their contrasting health care systems described earlier and the historical evolution of their public health institutions.

NEW YORK CITY: A STRATEGIC LOCAL ROLE IN HEALTH

New York City has roughly twice the national rate of recent immigrants and twice the rate of children and older persons living below the poverty line (Gusmano, Rodwin, and Cantor, 2007). Its health care system shares two key characteristics with the health system in the United States. First, it is characterized by fragmented employer-based private health insurance and public health insurance coverage for eligible beneficiary groups such as elderly or severely disabled people (Medicare), very poor people (Medicaid), children whose parents' income does not meet Medicaid eligibility standards (SCHIP), and veterans (Veterans Health Administration). Second, most primary care physicians and specialists work in private office-based fee-for-service practices with complex contracting arrangements among multiple payers, "preferred providers," and a continually changing organization of safety net providers who care for the uninsured.

In contrast, there are at least four ways in which New York City stands out in comparison with the broader health care system in the United States. First, it has a higher rate of uninsured residents (about 28% of the population in comparison with about 16% for the United States as a whole). Second, it has among the highest rates of persons 65 years or older who because of their recent immigrant status have not met the eligibility qualifications for Medicare. People in these population groups require a stronger safety net. The city's response to this need is the third respect in which it stands out from the nation as a whole: it has the largest public hospital system in the United States. The New York City Health and Hospitals Corporation (HHC) operates 11 of the city's 65 acute (short-stay) hospitals and is responsible for almost 20 percent of the total admissions to acute hospital beds. HHC is also responsible for delivering primary as well as specialist services in its outpatient departments, emergency rooms, and a network of health care centers. Finally, New York City stands out because its academic medical centers train the largest number of medical residents in the nation and because it is the home to one of the earliest and larger health maintenance organizations in the United States, the Health Insurance Plan of New York.

New York exercises a stronger local authority and responsibility for managing its local public health infrastructure than do our other two world cities. The New York City Department of Health and Mental Hygiene (DOHMH) is the oldest, largest, and strongest health department in the nation. Since its establishment in the 1860s in response to a cholera epidemic, much has changed in New York City, but DOHMH's mission to protect New Yorkers against infectious disease remains strong in light of the recent AIDS and tuberculosis epidemics, the West Nile and SARS scares, and post-9/11 concerns about the risks of bioterrorism, and more generally, emergency preparedness. From the 1990s on, it has exercised its authority in containing tuberculosis, regulating smoking, more generally integrating its public health surveillance system, and developing community health profiles that have led to targeting high-risk areas of the city.

Having recognized the need to improve public health infrastructure at the local level, in 1999 the Centers for Disease Control (CDC) awarded DOHMH a grant to improve the city's public health surveillance activities, including the capacity to develop community health profiles across the city's neighborhoods. Reinforced by the post-9/11 world, these activities led DOHMH to integrate its public health surveillance programs and redefine the nature of its collaboration and organizational relationships with the New York State Department of Health, the CDC, and other local agencies: the municipal HHC, the city's Office of Emergency Management, and of course, the fire and police departments. DOHMH also improved its relations with the physician community so that 80 percent of New York City physicians now communicate reportable diseases directly to the department. Perhaps most impressive are the systems of syndromic surveillance developed by DOHMH. For example, 60 percent of hospital emergency departments participate by monitoring their patients' diagnoses, and the Emergency Medical System monitors patterns of complaints for a sample of 911 calls.

Since 2000, DOHMH has also adopted new regulations and programs to combat a number of diseases whose consequences are reflected in our three indicators of access to health care: heart disease, colon cancer, and diabetes. In 2003, DOHMH formed the Citywide Colon Cancer Control Coalition to reduce colon cancer deaths through "advocacy, resource development, and policy initiatives" and by "facilitating communication between the health department and relevant stakeholders—health and social service organizations, academic institutions, governmental agencies and advocacy groups" (New York City, 2009). In 2006, it created a New York City A1C registry to help providers and patients improve diabetes care. Most laboratories in the city now report to DOHMH the results of A1C blood tests, which serve as an indicator of the average blood glucose control for the previous 2 to 3 months, for people who have diabetes. DOHMH issues quarterly reports from the A1C registry to health care providers in an effort to help them manage diabetes and reduce complications associated with it. Finally, DOHMH's recent bans on smoking in public buildings, restaurants, and bars and on artificial trans fats in city restaurants were both designed to reduce rates of heart disease, the leading cause of death among New Yorkers.

LONDON: LOCAL STRATEGIES FOR HEALTH IMPROVEMENT

Like New York City, London is a hub for so-called asylum-seekers in England, with the consequence that some of its boroughs rank among those with the highest levels of deprivation in England. In contrast to New York City, London's health care system is part of the National Health Service, which provides health care coverage to all legal residents. For the 33 boroughs of Greater London, NHS London is managed by the Strategic Health Authority (SHA), whose new mission is to ensure that all NHS services in London are world-class. The SHA oversees all 41 NHS hospitals, which are organized into 24 so-called acute trusts, 14 foundation trusts, and 3 mental health trusts (www.london.nhs.uk). The foundation trusts have the greatest latitude in managing their hospitals with respect to obtaining capital and hiring personnel. In addition, NHS hospitals contract with the private for-profit hospitals in London when waiting times for acute care procedures exceed current norms.

Along with oversight of NHS hospitals, the SHA oversees the delivery of primary care, which is organized by 31 primary care trusts. To obtain health services within the NHS, individuals must register with the PCTs covering their area of residence. Within the PCT, there is a choice of general practitioners who serve as gatekeepers to specialist services. In addition to providing primary care for patients, PCTs are increasingly being called upon to integrate a range of clinical prevention services and to contract for outreach services targeted at high-risk populations in their areas. This function highlights the complexity of coordinating primary care and public health functions. In this respect, London's public health institutions are, paradoxically, more fragmented than those in New York, even though many of them are supervised by the SHA. Whereas New York's DOHMH is responsible for the regulation of restaurants, in Greater London each of the 33 boroughs exercises this function independently.

Since 2000, the Greater London Authority has had an elected mayor. Some notable health-promotion efforts were associated with this change in citywide governance, highlighted by the city government's attempt to secure "healthy city" status from the WHO. The mayor, Ken Livingston, was given a powerful mandate to develop a public health agenda for Greater London. He placed significant emphasis on intersectoral interventions to improve health; among these were a biodiversity action plan and strategies directed toward improving transportation, municipal waste management, air quality, and ambient noise.

To implement this new approach, the mayor emphasized partnerships with the London Development Agency, the national government health agencies, and the city's voluntary sector. There is currently more public health monitoring and epidemiologic surveillance than ever before. Also, given the growing gap in London between a well-off majority and a poor minority, and the fact that nearly a quarter of the capital's population are ethnic minorities, much attention was paid to thinking about what policy interventions, programs, and monitoring activities should be developed to make Londoners healthier (London Health Commission, 2007).

Since 2002, the London Health Commission, which the mayor established in 2000, has published a *Health in London* report that tracks 10 health status indicators: life expectancy at birth, infant mortality, health self-assessments, citywide unemployment, unemployment among ethnic minorities, substandard housing, the domestic burglary rate, air quality (as measured by levels of NO_2 and PM_{10}), and road traffic casualties (London Health Commission, 2007). Since 2002 these reports have found steady increases in life expectancy at birth and education levels, improvements in housing and air quality, declines in infant mortality and road traffic casualties, and relative stability in rates of unemployment. Despite these positive developments, London still has health inequalities by ethnicity, social class, and neighborhood. The finding that "for every tube station along the Jubilee Line, from Westminster to the East End, Londoners living in these areas lose almost a year of expected life" serves as a dramatic illustration of these inequalities (London Health Commission, 2007: 19). The national and city governments have responded to this challenge by improving data collection, sharing data, and funding a host of special programs. London's Strategic Health Authority is working with PCTs to incorporate information about health disparities into their planning process. PCTs are expected to conduct health equity audits in which they examine access to specific services and geographic areas. Individual PCTs are implementing health education and care management efforts designed to improve health and tackle health inequalities (for example, by including nutrition and smoking cessation programs).

Local health agreements are another important mechanism used to address health inequalities and help overcome the fragmentation described above. These agreements set priorities for a local area based on agreement between the central government and the local authority. In London, special grants have been awarded to 10 boroughs with the goal of improving their performance with respect to the health status indicators noted earlier. Millions of pounds have been earmarked for physical activity programs, efforts to prevent teen pregnancies, chronic disease management models, healthy schools, smoking cessation programs, and support for vulnerable older persons and their caregivers, among other programs.

Alongside these important public health efforts the NHS is working to address long-standing problems in access to primary care services, which until recently was worse in London than in the rest of the country (Evandrou, 2006). Surveys suggest that since the late 1990s, access to general practitioners has improved "substantially" (Mayor of London, 2004). For example, Tower Hamlets, one of Inner London's more deprived boroughs, was cited by the mayor's office for significant improvement in access to general practitioners (Baldwin, 2005). Nevertheless, some PCTs are having difficulty achieving the national target of ensuring that patients can see a general practitioner within 48 hours (Campbell et al., 2005), and there are concerns about access to primary care for non-English-speaking patients (Camden Primary Care Trust, 2007).

PARIS: LOCAL HEALTH ROLES IN A CENTRALIZED STATE

Like New York City and London, Paris has seen its population become more heterogeneous with the rise of immigration from North Africa, Southeast Asia, and eastern Europe. Moreover, there are arrondissements of northeastern Paris, along with the department of Seine-Saint-Denis, with populations that have high rates of unemployment, low levels of education, and the income deprivation that accompanies these conditions. As in London, all legal residents in Paris are covered for health care under the French NHI Program. However, many vulnerable groups fall through the cracks, for as in New York City, and in contrast to London's NHS, responsibility for population health and delivery of primary care is not assigned to any entity comparable to a PCT. Despite a long tradition of centralized services in France, Paris illustrates the critical role of local authorities in assuming safety net responsibilities that have eluded its system of universal coverage under national health insurance.

In Paris, most public hospitals are managed by the Assistance Publique–Hôpitaux de Paris (AP-HP), an organization twice the size of the New York City Health and Hospitals Corporation. In contrast to New York's HHC, the hospitals of AP-HP dominate the hospital sector in Paris and its first ring, with more than one-half of acute hospital beds in Paris and a quasi-monopoly over hospital-based medical research and medical school training (Rodwin et al., 1992). The AP-HP hospitals include most of the best hospitals in Paris, and they serve not only the wealthiest members of society when they require the most specialized services, but also the poorest. Over the past decade, the private hospital sector has consolidated small proprietary hospitals and now presents some serious competition to AP-HP. Likewise, the increasing number of partnerships between public and private nonprofit hospitals represent a growing share of the Paris public hospital sector.

Like the New York City HHC, AP-HP operates major outpatient clinics. With respect to the provision of primary care, Paris comes closer to resembling New York City than London. Primary care is dominated by office-based, fee-for-service physicians. Approximately 50 percent of physicians do not accept NHI reimbursement as payment in full, and this figure can reach 80% for subspecialists. If patients choose to consult with physicians who require higher co-insurance payments, they are still eligible for some reimbursement under their complementary Medigap-type policies. If higher co-insurance payments constitute a financial barrier to access, patients can choose so-called sector 1 physicians, who accept NHI rates as payment in full. Some sector 1 physicians still work in private practice, but more often, patients will consult with them in hospital outpatient departments. If the normal co-insurance payments constitute a financial barrier to access, patients may also consult physicians at one of 50 health centers located in every arrondissement of the city, which serve as a safety net for all patients who fall through the cracks. Even after the extension of NHI in 2000 to the 3–4 percent of Parisians who were previously not covered, there are still illegal immigrants and others who make use of this network of safety net health centers.

Although there are relatively minor financial barriers to health care in Paris as compared with New York City, where 28 percent of the population is uninsured, there are nevertheless two local agencies that play an important role in the provision of health and social services for those who rely on safety net institutions. The first agency, the Paris Department of Social Action, Children's Services and Health (Direction de action sociale, de l'enfance et de la santé, or DASES) reflects the status of Paris as one of 95 departments in metropolitan France. The second agency, the Center for Social Action (Centre d'action sociale, or CAS) reflects the status of Paris as a local municipality (commune). DASES is under mayoral control but receives its funding from the central state; CAS is also under mayoral control but receives most of its funding from the Paris City Council. The administrative functions of these two agencies are not always clearly separated, but both play strategic roles with respect to the provision of health and social services to vulnerable populations: disadvantaged children, severely handicapped adults, drug abusers, the homeless, and all others who somehow fall through the cracks of the central welfare state. In addition, these agencies operate subsidized housing and many more programs for children and older persons. Despite these agencies, however, the creation of a host of national public health agencies (for AIDS, food safety, public health surveillance, and other programs) has kept the central government in a dominant role with respect to oversight of the health care system.

Paris authorities have taken strong measures since the Middle Ages to protect their citizens from health risks, including bubonic plague. Following the French Revolution, local responsibility for public health was explicitly defined. Despite a national commitment to the public hygiene movement in the nineteenth century, and France's identity as a strong centralized state, the central government has until recently played only a limited role in public health. At the time of the cholera epidemic (1837) and the outbreak of Spanish influenza (1918–19), the Paris Health Council was largely responsible for addressing the public response. Since World War II, a vast assortment of public agencies, operating at different territorial levels, have shared responsibility for the public health of Parisians.

For example, the Paris Prefecture, which is accountable to the Ministry of the Interior, is responsible for pest control and restaurant regulation. Regional and departmental agencies of the Ministry of Health are responsible for centrally designed public health programs. As noted earlier, the department of Paris has had its own agencies, DASES and CAS, to manage programs for children, older persons, and primary care for vulnerable Parisians. In addition, the Paris public hospital system (AP-HP) has initiated its own public health interventions including the analysis of public health information. Following the crisis over contaminated blood in the 1990s, the concern about AIDS and drug-resistant tuberculosis, and new awareness about the dangers of food poisoning, France established many new national agencies to safeguard public health. At the same time, DASES, CAS, AP-HP, and the voluntary sector have forged new alliances to protect public health and confront the rise of social inequalities, homelessness, delinquency among youth, and social exclusion.

With respect to disease surveillance and emergency preparedness, Paris resembles London, in that both would quickly be guided by national institutions in the event of a major disease outbreak. In contrast to New York City, there are no local institutions responsible for disease surveillance functions. For example, the French Institute for Public Health Surveillance (Institut de Veille Sanitaire)—the French equivalent of the U.S. CDC—and its local Interregional Epidemiology Units (Cellules Interrégionales d'Epidémiologie, CIRE) are responsible for coordinating epidemiologic surveillance for the greater Paris metropolitan region (Île de France). In the event of an emergency (e.g., an avian flu pandemic), key decisions would be made by the French Department of Homeland Security (the Ministère de l'Intérieur), and Paris would come under the responsibility of a designated zone connected to the Prefecture for the Police.

CONVERGENT TRENDS IN PUBLIC HEALTH INTERVENTION

Of the three cities studied here, New York City stands out because it has the largest share of population not covered under a national system that eliminates financial barriers to health care access. On the other hand, New York probably has the most sophisticated electronic surveillance systems, particularly for syndromic surveillance. Indeed, it is paradoxical that the health system characterized by the most severe access barriers to basic primary health care should be the one that is most prepared—from the perspective of surveillance—to move decisively in the event of an infectious disease epidemic.

Beyond these differences, however, and the contrasts in terms of public health organization, what is perhaps most striking is the emergence of convergent trends in public health intervention. In all three cities there is increasing awareness among public health leaders that the neighborhood is a critical spatial unit for targeted interventions to protect the population against risk factors for disease and to promote population health. In all three cities there are significant spatial disparities among neighborhoods in income, unemployment, educational attainment, housing, environmental conditions, and crime. These factors exercise profound effects on measures of differential population health status across city neighborhoods. They have important implications not only for how to target health protection and promotion programs, but also for how to improve emergency preparedness and communication with diverse urban populations.

Broader forces of globalization have no doubt reduced somewhat the contrast between New York and the other two cities over the past few decades. Consider an example of this phenomenon: the disparities in infant mortality rates among neighborhoods of these cities across two 5-year periods in the 1990s. There was a slight diminution of disparities within Manhattan and an increase in Paris and London, which suggests a possible "Manhattanization" of global cities (Rodwin and Neuberg, 2005). Another way of interpreting these data and many more of the health indicators compared is to distinguish between hard and "soft" global cities (Body-Gendrot, 1996). The softer ones tend to implement national programs that protect their most vulnerable populations from some of the forces of globalization. Thus, London and New York come out on the harder end, and Paris is distinctly softer. Beyond such a taxonomy, however, it is important to elaborate on the convergent trends in public health intervention which are increasingly targeted to "high-risk" neighborhoods.

New York City's Department of Health and Mental Hygiene recently placed special emphasis on the city's highest-risk neighborhoods in the South Bronx, east Brooklyn, and central Harlem. It has even engaged in a form of bureaucratic decentralization by opening up DOHMH offices in each of these three areas. In addition to establishing a DOHMH presence, the mission of these branch offices is to coordinate a range of formerly vertical public health programs and serve as advocates for improving community health.

In Paris and London, the areas of highest risk tend to be located along an east-west divide although the extent of residential segregation and social polarization is less severe than in New York. Both cities are also engaged in some targeting of higher-risk areas, but their approach is more influenced by national policies. In London, health "inequalities" have been the subject of many reports by the Department of Health and Social Security. As part of the effort to target health action zones at the national level, areas such as the boroughs of Tower Hamlet, Newham, Hackney, Camden-Islington, Lambeth, Southwark, and Lewisham have been selected for special attention. This involves borough-wide efforts to promote neighborhood "regeneration" through partnerships with social service agencies, housing improvement programs, and involvement by a variety of players ranging from local government, chambers of commerce, the police, and other voluntary organizations.

In Paris, the national urban targeting program (Politique de Ville) identified 11 neighborhoods, mostly on the basis of such criteria as high unemployment rates, to receive increased resources for community development. In these neighborhoods efforts involve less active participation of the public health community than is the case in London. Rather than formulating explicit health improvement programs from which relations to other agencies radiate, this approach subsumes public health concerns within the broader net of social inclusion and neighborhood regeneration programs. But increasingly, there are discussions among city authorities about how to target limited resources to areas of the city in the greatest need. The areas selected by the Politique de Ville are spread out across all of Paris, but 5 of the 11 projects are concentrated in the 18th and 20th arrondissements (in neighborhoods such as the Goutte-d'Or, Barbes, Belleville, and Chateau Rouge) in the northeast of Paris and parts of the 13th arrondissement in the southeast.

How to Compare Health Systems in World Cities?

Because the health care systems in the United States, France, and England differ in their financing, provider payment mechanisms, and delivery system organization, efforts to understand the implications of these differences for access to care are complicated. Moreover, the populations of these three nations differ in size, age, racial and ethnic makeup, and socioeconomic status. These countries also differ in levels of medical resources (e.g., density of physicians, hospital beds, and medical technologies). These differences make it exceedingly difficult to isolate the influence of the health care system characteristics that we have described on access to health care. But concentrating on cities and comparing access to health care among and within these cities helps to overcome this problem because they have many more features in common than do their respective nations. By reducing the population, economic, and health care resource differences, one can more easily identify the contributions of health care financing and organization policies on access to health care services.*

To accomplish our goal of comparing access to care among these cities, we begin with one of the first problems to emerge in any comparative inquiry: how to define the relevant units of analysis. When the United

* This section draws on material presented in Rodwin and Gusmano (2006b).

Nations and other international organizations classify our three cities, they often refer to the entire New York Metropolitan Region, Île de France (which includes Paris and its two surrounding rings), or the Greater London Region. But we do not regard these vast agglomerations as appropriate geographic units for comparing health care in world cities. The image of world cities is usually rooted in their historical and spatial development around an urban core. Moreover, their urban cores are most directly connected to their functions as centers of "command and control" in the global economy and to their centrality in the world of culture, education, and the media.

THE URBAN CORE AS A UNIT OF ANALYSIS

In defining the urban core of New York City, Paris, and London, our initial studies were guided by six criteria: (1) historic and spatial development; (2) population size; (3) population density; (4) mix of high- and low-income populations; (5) spatial distribution of employment and commuter patterns; and (6) density of health system resources (hospital beds and physicians). These are summarized under the headings below.

Development and Population
With respect to spatial development, Manhattan, Paris, and Inner London represent the historic centers from which these metropolitan regions grew. Their populations range from 1.5 to 2.6 million (Table 2.2). Manhattan and Paris are similar in terms of density—66,000 versus 53,000 inhabitants per square mile—with both having almost twice the population density of Inner London.

Social and Economic Characteristics of the Population
The urban cores of the three cities combine a mix of high- and low-income populations, though there are substantial differences with regard to the degree of economic inequality within these cities. The poverty rate, defined as the percentage of households with incomes below one-half of the median, is almost twice as high in Manhattan (28.5%) as in Paris (12.8%). The poverty level for Manhattan, and New York City as a whole, is defined as the percentage of households with incomes below one-half

TABLE 2.2. Population characteristics of urban cores and their countries

City/country	Total population (millions)	% of population		
		>65 years of age	Foreign-born	Nonwhite
Manhattan	1.5	13.9	28.4	53.1
Paris	2.1	15.4	22.7	NA
Inner London	2.6	11	33.7	34.3
United States	281	12.6	10.4	24.9
France	57.3	16.1	5.6	NA
England	52	15.9	8.3	8

DATA SOURCES: Manhattan and United States—U.S. Census, 2000; Paris and France—French Census, 1999; London and England—National Office of Statistics, UK, 2001.

of Manhattan median income; for Paris and its agglomeration (a slightly larger area than Paris and its first ring) it is measured as the percentage of households with incomes below one-half of the median income. Data for both cities refer to pretax income; for Manhattan, pretax income includes Social Security payments and welfare payments but does not include other transfer payments (e.g., food stamps).

Although it is not possible to obtain household data for the United Kingdom, a comparison of occupational and class categories defined by the census may be used as a proxy for income. Although these data are not comparable to the income figures for Manhattan and Paris, they do allow us to observe a similar pattern in all three cities—poverty rates in the urban core are slightly higher than in their first rings. In the Paris agglomeration, the poverty rate is 10.2 percent; in New York it is 25.6 percent. In Greater London the share of lower "classes" is 14.9 percent, as opposed to 17 percent in Inner London.

With the exception of New York, a similar pattern holds for the percentage of foreign-born populations. Inner London has the highest share of foreign-born (33.7%), followed by Manhattan (28.4%) and Paris (22.7%). In Paris and Inner London this population is higher than in the first ring, but the percentage of foreign-born population in Manhattan is lower than in the surrounding boroughs. All three urban cores are significantly more diverse, in terms of the percentage of foreign-born, than their respective nations.

It is against the law to collect data on race or ethnicity in France, but we are able to compare the percentage of the population that is "non-white" in the United States and Manhattan to that of England and Inner London. It is clear that Manhattan and Inner London are also more alike than their respective nations with regard to ethnic diversity.

The percentage of single-parent families is much higher in Manhattan (22.8%) than in Paris (14.7%) or Inner London (9.8%). Birth rates are highest in Inner London (64.6) and roughly the same in Manhattan and Paris (around 48 per 1,000 females aged 15-45).

The health status of residents in these three world cities appears to be the same as or better than the health status of those living in their nations as a whole. Table 2.3 shows infant mortality rates as well as life expectancy at birth and at age 65 for men and women in the three cities and countries. Older persons in Paris and New York live longer than their counterparts in the two nations as a whole. Of the three cities, New York

TABLE 2.3. Infant mortality rate and life expectancy in world cities and their countries

City/country	Infant mortality rate	Life expectancy at birth (years)		Life expectancy at age 65 (years)	
		Males	Females	Males	Females
New York City	6.2	74.5 (2000)	80.2 (2000)	17.0 (2000)	20.1 (2000)
Paris	4.0[a]	77.6[b] (2002)	83.1[b] (2002)	17.7 (1999)	21.7 (1999)
Greater London	5.4	76.1 (2000–2004)	80.9 (2000–2004)	15.6 (1997–99)	19.2 (1997–99)
United States	7.0 (2002)	74.3 (2000)	79.7 (2000)	16.3 (2000)	19.2 (2000)
France	4.1	77.1 (2002)	83.4 (2002)	16.5 (1999)	21.0 (1999)
England	5.3 (2003)	76.3[c] (2000–2004)	80.8[c] (2000–2004)	15.7 (1999–2001)	18.9 (1997–99)

DATA SOURCES: New York City and United States—National Center for Health Statistics/ Centers for Disease Control; Paris and France—Institut National de la Statistique et des Etudes Economiques (INSEE), Observatoire Régional de la Santé de l'Île de France; London and England—Office of National Statistics, London Health Observatory.

[a] For Paris and first ring.
[b] For Paris only.
[c] For England only.

has the highest infant mortality rate and lowest life expectancy at birth and at 65, while the infant mortality rate is lowest and life expectancy is highest in Paris.

Most of these differences—in health status, poverty rates, birth rates, and family structure—reflect national patterns and policies with regard to income maintenance and immigration. Other differences—population density and percentage of the older old—are distinctive urban characteristics.

Concentrated Centers of Employment

All three urban cores have economies based on services and information, which are closely tied to national and international transactions. They are also centers of culture, media, government, and international organizations. All three function as employment centers that attract large numbers of commuters. Approximately one-third of the first ring's employed labor force commute to Manhattan, Paris, and Inner London every day (Rodwin and Gusmano, 2006a).

Centers of Medical Excellence

Manhattan, Paris, and Inner London are each centers of medical excellence within their nations. Each of the three urban areas has a much higher density of physicians than their first ring or their nations as a whole (Table 2.4). The ratio of physician density between the core and the first ring is higher for Manhattan (4.0) than for Inner London (3.6) or Paris (2.3).

Although these three urban cores are much more alike than are their nations with regard to the number of practicing physicians, there are important differences among them as well. For example, they differ in the balance among primary care and specialist physicians. In terms of numbers of general practitioners, the primary care system is clearly much stronger in Paris and Inner London than it is in Manhattan. In Manhattan, less than 30 percent of all physicians are in primary care, but in Inner London and Paris half are in primary care.

All three urban cores have higher levels of acute care hospital beds than their first rings or their respective nations. Manhattan and Inner London have 2.7 and 2.6 times as many beds as their first rings; Paris has 1.8 times as many. These ratios indicate the concentration of acute hospital beds including those among large university teaching hospitals in all of the central cores (see Table 2.4).

TABLE 2.4. Densities of physicians and acute care hospital beds

City/country	No. of physicians per 10,000 persons	No. of acute care hospital beds per 1,000 persons
New York City (2000/2002)		
Urban core	75.4	7.0
First ring	18.8	2.6
Ratio[a]	4.0	2.7
Paris Region (2002/2001)		
Urban core	84.6	7.0
First ring	37.0	3.9
Ratio[a]	2.3	1.8
Greater London (1999/2000)		
Urban core	36.9	3.7
First ring	10.3	1.4
Ratio[a]	3.6	2.6
United States	27	3.1
France	30	4.3
England	20	2.2

DATA SOURCES: For physicians: New York City—New York State Department of Health, 1995; Paris—Ministère de l'Emploi et de la Solidarité, Service des Statistiques des Études et des Systèmes d'Information (SESI), repertoire ADELI au 1er janvier 98; London—London Health Observatory, 2000.

For hospital beds: New York City and United States—Health Care Annual, United Hospital Fund; Paris and France—Direction Régionale des Affaires Sanitaires et Sociales; London—London Health Observatory, 2000; England—Department of Health and Social Security.

[a] Ratio = urban core / first ring

Summary

Paris—a city of 2.1 million all living within the nineteenth-century walls and the peripheral freeway that surrounds its 20 arrondissements—was the prototypical "urban core" against which we selected comparable urban cores for New York and London. The population of Paris and its land area (105 square kilometers) is minuscule in comparison to Greater London's 7.9 million people and 1,590 square kilometers and to New York City's 8 million people and 826 square kilometers. Rather, it is comparable to the urban core of these cities. For New York City, this is Manhattan with its 1.5 million people; for London, it is the 14 boroughs known as "Inner London," with a population of 2.7 million.

Although there are important differences among them, these three urban cores are in many respects more alike than their respective nations. They are comparable in terms of the size, age, and diversity of the population. All three play similar roles in the global economy and have a concentration of financial and medical resources. Because they have so much in common, comparing access to primary and specialty health care in these three "world cities" provides unique insight into the ways that health system differences contribute to difference in access. We begin this inquiry in Chapter 3 with a comparison of "avoidable mortality" within and among these urban cores and their nations.

CHAPTER THREE

Overall Performance of the Health System

Avoidable Mortality

O UR HEALTH STATUS may depend on behavior and lifestyle, the environment in which we live, and our genes more than on the health care we receive, but for people with illness for which treatment exists, access to timely and effective health care is crucial. Health services can reduce rates of premature mortality due to certain conditions, such as leukemia, breast cancer, and a host of infectious diseases. If the rate of premature mortality due to these conditions—so-called avoidable mortality—is higher, for example, in Manhattan than in Paris, this suggests that Manhattanites face greater barriers to life-prolonging health services. Because we are concerned with the degree to which Manhattan, Paris, and Inner London provide access to health care for people who need it, comparing avoidable mortality among as well as within these cities serves as an important indicator of overall performance of the health system.

This chapter compares rates of avoidable mortality in our three nations and their world cities. In addition, we examine the association between avoidable mortality and neighborhood income within the cities. For each area, we measure the correlation between the place of residence and age- and gender-adjusted total mortality and avoidable mortality rates for two time periods, 1988–1990 and 1998–2000. To assess the geographic distribution of access to health care within each city, we rely on regression models that estimate the association of neighborhood income with avoidable mortality.

As we expected, France has the lowest rate of total mortality. The United States has a higher total mortality rate, but its avoidable mortality rate is similar to that of England. Among the cities, rates of avoidable mortality are lowest in Paris and highest in Inner London. Avoidable mortality rates are higher in poor neighborhoods of all three cities; but only in Manhattan is there a significant correlation between avoidable mortality and the median household income of the neighborhood in which the decedents resided. Disparities in avoidable mortality are greatest in Manhattan.

Why Is It Useful to Examine Avoidable Deaths?

In comparison with other wealthy nations, the United States has poor health status (OECD, 2005). Indeed, a recent comparison of England and the United States indicates that Americans have inferior health status compared with the English (Banks et al., 2006). Banks, Marmot, and co-authors conducted an ingenious study comparing the health of middle-aged white residents of England and the United States. According to their survey data, white Americans age 55 to 64 years have higher rates of diabetes, high blood pressure, heart disease, heart attack, stroke, lung disease, and cancer than their English counterparts.

While such findings are important, most reported health indicators fail to distinguish between the determinants of population health not directly related to health care (e.g., poverty, lifestyle, or education), so their use in evaluating the performance of the health system is limited (WHO, 2006). An alternative approach, as we try to learn from international experience, is to compare selected causes of mortality that have been linked more directly to health care system performance. By conducting such an analysis across and within Manhattan, Paris, and Inner London, our comparison of avoidable mortality represents a first step in assessing the influence of health systems on population health and access to health care.

The concept of avoidable mortality developed by Rutstein et al. (1976) assumes that an avoidable death signals evidence of health system failure. Although the analysis of avoidable mortality is only one dimension of health system performance, it has been widely adopted in Europe (Holland, 1997). The concept of avoidable mortality also assumes that health care should be able to prevent premature death from diseases amenable to a combination of different interventions, including health education, screening, and health care services. Premature death due to breast, colorectal, and skin cancer, for example, can be reduced dramatically through the use of screening and early detection (Hakama et al., 1997; Peto et al.,

2004; Sante et al., 2003; Tabar et al., 1992). Similarly, maternal death can be prevented through the use of antibiotics, safe blood transfusions, and access to emergency surgical care (Rosenfield and Figdor, 2001; Rosenfield and Maine, 1985).

More recently, avoidable mortality has been refined by differentiating deaths from conditions that are amenable to health care interventions from those that could be prevented by broader health promotion policies such as improving highway safety, reducing medical errors, or altering health behaviors (Berwick, 2005; Chassin et al., 1998). Some have further categorized each cause of avoidable mortality with respect to conventional concepts of disease prevention as primary, secondary, or tertiary (Tobias and Jackson, 2001).

According to the U.S. Preventive Services Task Force, primary prevention services are those "provided to prevent the onset of a targeted condition" (U.S. Preventive Services Task Force, 1996: xli). These include immunizations, health education, and counseling to encourage the adoption and maintenance of healthy lifestyles. For example, the American Heart Association encourages physicians to reinforce public health messages regarding "the avoidance of tobacco, healthy dietary patterns, weight control, and regular, appropriate exercise" (AHA, 2002: 388). Similarly, the Advisory Committee on Immunization Practices (ACIP), the U.S. Centers for Disease Control (CDC), the European Union Geriatric Medical Society (EUGMS), the International Association of Geriatrics and Gerontology–European Region (IAGG-ER), and the World Health Organization (WHO) have all called for improving rates of influenza and pneumococcal vaccination among persons 50 or older to reduce rates of hospitalization and premature mortality (Gusmano and Michel, 2009).

Secondary prevention identifies and treats "asymptomatic persons who have already developed risk factors or preclinical disease but in whom the condition is not clinically apparent" (U.S. Preventive Services Task Force, 1996: xli). These include screening tests during the latency period for conditions such as hyperlipidemia and hypertension, precursors of heart disease and stroke, or breast and prostate cancer. Recent comparisons of the United States and Europe suggest that higher breast cancer survival rates for women in the United States can be attributed, in part, to early detection and the more aggressive use of mammography (Sante et al., 2003).

In contrast, "tertiary" prevention involves care of a diagnosed disease with efforts to prevent disease-related complications. One example is the use of aspirin, statins, and anti-hypertensive therapy (beta blockers, and angiotensin-converting enzyme inhibitors) for patients diagnosed with ischemic heart disease (IHD) (Unal, Critchley, and Capewell, 2005).

In France, avoidable mortality has been used to account for gender disparities in premature mortality, with an emphasis on conditions closely related to risk behavior. For example, Lefèvre and colleagues analyze gender disparities in premature mortality–related alcohol abuse, tobacco abuse, and dangerous driving. They conclude that gender differences in rates of avoidable mortality call for more primary prevention (Lefèvre et al., 2004). A concept of avoidable mortality, referring to conditions amenable to health care rather than deaths related to risky behavior, had not previously been applied to a study of Paris.

Despite the strengths described above, analysis of avoidable mortality as an indicator of access to health care across these three systems is limited because it is difficult to disentangle the relative importance of primary, secondary, and tertiary prevention and therapeutic care. Most of the deaths that are captured by the definition of avoidable mortality are influenced by more than one aspect of the health care system. People who die prematurely from cancer or IHD may not have benefited from disease prevention service, or may have been engaged in risky behavior, or, once they were diagnosed with IHD or cancer, may not have received appropriate treatment.

Beyond the issue of attributing changes in rates of avoidable mortality to specific interventions, we recognize that mortality is an incomplete measure of access to timely and effective health care services. Yet, in this era of privacy concerns, reliable population-level, disease-specific morbidity data are rarely available and can only reflect patients who are already involved in the health care system and not all of those in need of care. There are surveys that provide some useful information, but the samples are usually too small to allow us to investigate the influence of local factors on health status or the use of health services.

We relied on vital statistics publications derived from death certificates to determine the cause of death. The "main cause of death" was used in our rate calculations, an approach consistent with that of others using these data. We acknowledge that only one "cause" can be given, even for persons with multiple health problems. In some circumstances it is difficult to know the precise cause of death. Using vital statistics data always carries the risk that information may be unreliable for certain conditions where the cause of death is poorly known, for multiple conditions, or where conditions carry a social stigma. Moreover, as Nolte and McKee (2003: 328) explain, "For many conditions, death is the final event in a complex chain of processes that involve issues related to underlying social and economic factors, lifestyles, and preventive and curative health care." Avoidable mortality is more closely related to the health care system, but our capacity to identify the precise contribution of medical services is limited.

In addition, our ability to compare the assignment of causes of death is always a concern. If deaths are misclassified more commonly in one geographic area than in another, the results could be biased. However, the inclusion of a large group of causes of death makes this problem less likely.

All of these limitations must be weighed against the advantages of using mortality statistics in assessing population health. These advantages include their widespread availability and the fact that death is obviously a clearly defined event. Although physician diagnostic habits and preferences could represent another source of bias, differences in avoidable deaths do persist among regions even after controlling for disease incidence (Treurniet et al., 1999).

Our comparison of avoidable deaths in Manhattan, Paris, and Inner London allows us not only to explore the extent to which their respective health systems affect access to health care but also to highlight possible opportunities for reducing premature mortality across and within these cities. We provide some initial conclusions about the characteristics of these health care systems that may contribute to these differences and discuss the more detailed geographic and clinical-level data needed to identify effective specific health care interventions.

Population Health and Avoidable Deaths

A host of earlier studies suggests that health care contributes little to declines in mortality and the improvement of population health (Cochrane, St. Leger, and Moore, 1978; McKeown, 1979; McKinlay and McKinlay,

1977) and that some medical interventions are damaging to health (Illich, 1976). Nevertheless, effective therapies for a variety of conditions have been developed since the mid-twentieth century (Fogel, 2000), and many scholars who emphasize the importance of social determinants recognize that medical care can prolong life "after some serious diseases" (Wilkinson and Marmot, 2003). Mackenbach examined the effects of antibiotics on infectious diseases, advances in surgical and anesthetic techniques on appendicitis and gall bladder disease, and ante- and perinatal care on infant mortality for 1875 to 1970 in the Netherlands and concluded that a 5 to 18.5 percent decline in mortality could be attributed to improved health care (Mackenbach, 1996). A study seeking to explain the decline in coronary heart disease mortality in England between 1981 and 2000 attributed 42 percent of the decrease to medical treatment of individuals and 58 percent to a reduction in population risk factors, primarily smoking (Unal, Critchley, and Capewell, 2004). Nolte and McKee published an extensive review of the literature on avoidable mortality and conclude that health care has made an appreciable difference to population health although the rate varies among countries (Nolte and McKee, 2003, 2004). For example, they found that in 1998, France had a standardized rate of avoidable mortality of 75 per 100,000, but the United Kingdom had a rate of 134 per 100,000.

The definition of avoidable mortality has evolved over the past several decades as the ability of medical care to increase life expectancy has improved. Cross-national analysis of trends in avoidable mortality in Europe indicate that avoidable deaths declined much faster over the last two decades than other causes of mortality. This result lends further credence to the validity of avoidable mortality as an indicator for the effectiveness of public health interventions and medical care (Treurniet, Boshuizen, and Harteloh, 2004).

We based our selection of causes of death considered avoidable (see the Appendix) on work by Nolte and McKee (2004), who presented a detailed justification for the diagnoses they chose. Their list is, in turn, a modification of the work of Tobias and Jackson (2001), Mackenbach (1996), and Charlton et al. (1986). Needless to say, few conditions are entirely amenable, or not amenable, to health care, and as medical therapies improve, even more deaths may be classified as avoidable. Our list of "avoidable" causes of death differs from that employed by others in that we eliminate those causes usually restricted to people younger than 15 years of age (intestinal infections, whooping cough, measles, respiratory diseases other than pneumonia and influenza), all of which are relatively uncommon as causes of death. Because we compared infant mortality across our world cities in Chapter 2, our analysis of avoidable deaths starts at one year. The upper age limit, because the definition of avoidable mortality includes the concept of premature death, was set at 75 years. The likelihood that a condition will be amenable to intervention becomes increasingly questionable at older ages. Furthermore, at older ages there is a higher probability of serious co-morbidities. Death certificates record only a single cause of death, so they are less reliable for older persons (Nolte and McKee, 2003). While any upper age limit for avoidable mortality is arbitrary, the age of 75 is only slightly below life expectancy at birth in France, England, and the United States. We also include all deaths from diabetes mellitus, leukemia, and malignancy of the cervix and body of the uterus. For the sake of simplicity—and because most health care providers we surveyed believe that the ability to prevent deaths from these illnesses among those 75 years or younger is contingent on disease process, not age—we use this upper age limit for all conditions.

IHD is included in our definition, but because this diagnosis affects such large numbers of people, it may obscure the contribution of some other causes of avoidable mortality. In response to this concern, we adopt the approach suggested by Nolte and McKee (2003) by presenting avoidable mortality with only half of the deaths from IHD included in the definition. It is clear that primary prevention contributes significantly to reductions in mortality from IHD. In New York, for example, antismoking efforts during the past decade have produced dramatic decreases in rates of smoking, a major contributor to the development of IHD.

As we mentioned in Chapter 1, recent studies suggest that secondary prevention and the use of tertiary care contribute to lower mortality as well (Unal, Critchley, and Capewell, 2005). Including half of the deaths from IHD is arbitrary, but the latest available evidence suggests this is a reasonable estimate (Bots and Grobbee, 1996; Capewell, Morrison, and McMurrey, 1999; Unal, Critchley, and Capewell, 2004, 2005). An extensive literature indicates that the impact of therapy is substantial, such that a considerable proportion of deaths due to IHD are amenable at some level of care (Capewell, Morrison, and McMurrey, 1999, 2000; Hunink et al., 1997; see our Appendix for additional details).

Country, City, and Neighborhood Differences

We use chi square testing to determine statistical significance for area-level differences. To test the null hypothesis that mortality and area of residence are independent, we relied on a variable, "living," consisting of the category "survivors," a variable "area" consisting of the categories "United States," "England," and "France" (or "Manhattan," "Inner London," and "Paris"), and "dies unavoidably" and "dies avoidably" for either 1988–1990 or 1998–2000. If rejected, then the alternative hypothesis is that mortality and area of residence are significantly associated.

One of the benefits of extending national comparisons of these indicators with city-level comparisons is the ability to examine the extent to which there are geographic disparities in access to health care services. We estimated the relationship between a neighborhood-level income indicator and the percentage of avoidable deaths during the period 1998 to 2000, using ordinary least squares regression. Because avoidable deaths are a rare occurrence and a nonnegative count variable, and exhibit greater variation than in a true Poisson process, we used a negative binomial regression model to assess the influence of neighborhood income on the rate of avoidable mortality. The number of deaths is the "response," the population less than 75 years of age is the "exposure," and the income-related indicator is the explanatory variable. We report not the estimate of the underlying coefficient of the income variable but the exponential of the estimate, the estimated incident rate ratio. This is the ratio of the value of the avoidable mortality rate in the low-income (or high-deprivation) areas to that of the rest of the city. If the incident rate ratio is 1, there is no difference in mortality between low-income areas and the remainder of the city. Alternatively, if the incident ratio is greater than 1, the low-income areas have higher avoidable mortality rates than the remainder of the city.

For all national and city-level units of analysis, the age- and sex-adjusted total and avoidable mortality rates decreased over the decade studied (Table 3.1). During the two time periods, France has the lowest overall total mortality and avoidable mortality rates. The total mortality rate for England is lower than the rate for the United States in both time

TABLE 3.1. Total and avoidable mortality rates in urban cores and countries, 1988–1990 and 1998–2000

City/country	1988–1990 average			1998–2000 average		
	Total (N)	Avoidable, with 50% IHD deaths (N)	Avoidable, excluding all IHD (N)	Total (N)	Avoidable, with 50% IHD deaths (N)	Avoidable, excluding all IHD (N)
Manhattan	5.64 (8,260)	1.47 (2,125)	1.10 (1,593)	3.69 (5,281)	1.18 (1,686)	0.91 (1,300)
Paris	3.68 (7,637)	0.78 (1,614)	0.66 (1,370)	2.94 (5,809)	0.66 (1,306)	0.58 (1,151)
Inner London	4.95 (11,969)	1.70 (4,042)	1.14 (2,521)	4.32 (11,200)	1.49 (3,868)	1.07 (2,782)
United States	4.54 (1,053,637)	1.38 (319,409)	0.95 (220,061)	4.00 (1,017,937)	1.19 (302,175)	0.86 (218,316)
France	3.72 (193,538)	0.87 (45,075)	0.71 (37,020)	3.26 (175,876)	0.76 (40,815)	0.64 (34,644)
England	4.26 (186,169)	1.52 (66,723)	0.94 (41,158)	3.57 (169,490)	1.23 (58,407)	0.85 (40,352)

NOTE: Rates for ages 1–74 per 1,000 population. Avoidable mortality rates are adjusted for age and gender.

periods, but rates of avoidable mortality exceed that of the United States when half of deaths due to IHD are included. If IHD is excluded from the definition, England and the United States have avoidable mortality rates that are nearly identical.

Similarly, Paris has the lowest total mortality and avoidable mortality rates, while Manhattan fares better than Inner London for avoidable mortality. We did conduct a sensitivity analysis in which we included all deaths from IHD in the definition of avoidable mortality, but this did not change the results: even in this case, the rates of avoidable mortality are lowest in Paris and highest in Inner London.

The differences between France, the United States, and the urban cores of their world cities are larger for avoidable mortality than for total mortality. The total mortality rate for England is lower than in the United States. When we compare avoidable mortality, however, England and Inner London had higher rates than the United States and Manhattan. When we compare Inner London and Manhattan, the avoidable mortality rates for Inner London are higher for all of the definitions we examined. For total mortality, Manhattan also has a lower rate than Inner London in the recent time period. Manhattan previously had a higher total mortality rate.

In all three nations and urban cores, IHD was the largest single cause of avoidable mortality. In France and England, as well as in Paris and Inner London, the second largest category of avoidable mortality was cancer of the colon, rectum, breast, or cervix, followed by premature deaths attributed to hypertension and stroke. In the United States and Manhattan, this is reversed, with deaths from hypertension and stroke exceeding the malignancies listed above. Influenza, asthma and bronchitis, and diabetes represent the next largest causes in all areas.

The rates of avoidable mortality declined in all three urban cores over the 1988–1990 and the 1998–2000 periods, but Manhattan experienced the greatest decline in the rate of avoidable mortality (20%) in comparison with Paris (16%) and Inner London (13%). Once again, the results were comparable when we include all IHD deaths in the definition of avoidable mortality. The chi square test, based on numbers of avoidable and unavoidable deaths, indicates that the differences we observe among these nations and cities are statistically significant (Table 3.2).

TABLE 3.2. Number of avoidable and unavoidable deaths and survivors in urban cores and countries, 1988–1990 and 1998–2000

	Avoidable deaths	"Unavoidable deaths"	Survivors
	1988–1990		
Manhattan	2,027	5,763	1,374,164
Paris	1,530	5,710	1,963,143
London	4,042	7,927	2,385,841
Chi square=1,104.43, 4 degrees of freedom*			
United States	319,409	734,228	230,831,430
France	45,075	148,464	51,802,436
England	66,723	119,446	43,528,331
Chi square=13,234.26, 4 degrees of freedom*			
	1998–2000		
Manhattan	1,686	3,594	1,427,294
Paris	1,306	4,503	1,968,928
London	3,868	7,332	2,582,254
Chi square=812.97, 4 degrees of freedom*			
United States	302,175	715,762	253,247,063
France	40,815	135,060	53,714,086
England	58,407	111,084	47,257,610
Chi square=12,090.56, 4 degrees of freedom*			

* Chi square significant at the .001 level

Neighborhood Disparities in Preventable Death

The notion that neighborhood characteristics, including the "built" or physical environment, influence population health is now well established in the public health literature (Cohen et al., 2003; Davey Smith et al., 1998; LaVeist and Wallace, 2000; Northridge and Sclar, 2003). Previous studies of all three health care systems have also found evidence of geographic disparities in access to health care (Chaix et al., 2005; Oliver, Healey, and Le Grand, 2002; Roos and Mustard, 1997). For example, one recent survey found that older persons listed a lack of transportation as one of the major barriers to seeing a physician (Fitzpatrick et al., 2004). The problem is most pronounced in the United States, where race-based residential segregation and the geographic concentration of poverty among blacks and other minority groups is often reflected in significant geographic disparities in access to health care services (Weisz and Gusmano, 2006).

To estimate the relationship between neighborhood-level income and avoidable mortality, we use a similar measure of average pretax household income by neighborhood subunit for Manhattan and Paris. Because household income data are not available in the United Kingdom, for London we use the deprivation index in place of a direct income measure.* Using income and the deprivation index as explanatory variables in the model would make London and the other two cities difficult to compare. As in our previous analysis of infant mortality and income (Rodwin and Neuberg, 2005), we used income and the deprivation index to define an indicator variable that was used as the explanatory variable in the model. For Manhattan and Paris, we set income equal to 1 if a neighborhood was in the lowest income quartile (Manhattan has three neighborhoods in lowest quartile; Paris, five). For London we let income equal 1 for each of the four boroughs in the highest deprivation quartile; for all other neighborhoods we let income equal 0. If the deprivation index in London captures the four lowest-income neighborhoods in the most-deprived quartile, our combination of income and deprivation indicators selects the lowest income quartile neighborhoods for the three urban cores.

When we estimated the relationship between neighborhood-level income and percentage of avoidable mortality during the period 1998 to 2000 using ordinary least squares regression, we found a correlation in Manhattan at the 1 percent level of significance but no significant correlation in Paris or London at the 5 percent level (Table 3.3). Negative binomial regression results reveal that residence in a low-income neighborhood is always significantly associated with increased avoidable mortality rates and that the incident rate ratio is greatest in Manhattan, followed by Inner London, and is lowest in Paris.

* The derivation of the deprivation index is available at www.communities.gov.uk/communities/neighbourhoodrenewal/deprivation.

TABLE 3.3. Regression results for the number of avoidable deaths, using total deaths and lowest-income-quartile neighborhoods as independent variables, 1998–2000

	Manhattan[a]			Paris[b]			Inner London[c]		
R^2	.941			.987			.542		
					ANOVA				
F	72.408			667.962			6.510		
(Sig)	(.000)			(.000)			(.014)		
Df	11			19			13		
					Coefficients				
	B	t	Sig	B	T	Sig	B	t	Sig
(Constant)	6,925.194	.376	.716	1,096.902	.386	.704	73,439.734	.951	.362
Total no. of deaths	162.695	8.354	.000	127.061	29.722	.000	146.922	3.319	.007
Neighborhood with lowest quartile income	68,461.511	3.661	.005*	8,545.365	2.084	.053	28,220.435	.487	.636

[a] Incident rate ratio (IRR) = 1.66; SE = .302; Z stat = 2.81; P value = 0.005
[b] IRR = 1.06; SE = .098; Z stat = 3.01; P value = 0.003
[c] IRR = 1.19; SE = .077; Z stat = 2.81; P value = 0.005
* Significant at p < .05 level

The Policy Context for Interpreting Avoidable Mortality

The United States does not provide universal access to health care; as a consequence, more than 46 million Americans do not have health insurance. In Manhattan, about 24 percent of the population is uninsured (Sandman, Schoen, and DesRoches, 1998), and our comparison of avoidable hospital conditions in Manhattan and Paris (Chapter 4) suggests that Manhattanites have poorer access to primary health care than do Parisians, who face few financial barriers to care and are surrounded by a high concentration of health services.

Like residents of Paris, residents of Inner London do not have significant financial barriers to health care, but the density of hospital beds and doctors in Inner London is lower than in the two other urban cores (Chapter 2). Furthermore, greater restrictions placed by the NHS on the availability of some specialty services may influence the rate of avoidable mortality. For example, in comparison with France and the United States, the NHS provides fewer revascularizations for patients with IHD and less access to chemotherapy for patients with cancer. Even though residents of Inner London have greater access to revascularization than the rest of England, the use of these services is clearly much lower than in the other urban cores (Chapter 5).

Despite these important national differences, all three of these countries and cities have launched aggressive primary and secondary prevention efforts, including screening programs for a variety of diseases. The NHS Breast Screening Program, created by the Department of Health in 1988, was expanded in 1990 to cover the entire nation; in 2000, an analysis concluded that the program had lowered mortality rates from breast cancer among women age 55–69 (*BMJ*, 2000). The NHS Cervical Screening Program, established in 1988, screens almost 4 million women in England each year. This program is credited with reducing the cervical cancer mortality rate among women younger than 35 (Peto et al., 2004).

Although a host of successful screening programs for cancer were implemented at the district level in France during the 1990s, until recently mass cancer screening programs have been more limited there than in England. In 2003, President Chirac renewed the French National Cancer

Control Plan, which allocated funds for the acceleration of mass screening programs for breast, cervical, and colorectal cancer.

The U.S. Department of Health and Human Services and the New York City Department of Health and Mental Hygiene have also launched aggressive health promotion campaigns designed to encourage early detection and screening for a host of diseases, including breast, cervical, and colon and rectal cancer and heart disease. Since the late 1980s, New York City's public health efforts have resulted in greater declines in infant mortality and tuberculosis than have those in London or Paris (Rodwin and Gusmano, 2002). As a result, although we had anticipated that the overall rate of avoidable mortality would remain highest in Manhattan, we did expect over the two time periods that there would be a larger decline in rates of avoidable mortality in Manhattan than in the other urban cores.

Can we attribute differences in avoidable mortality to differences among health systems? There is a much greater difference between the United States and France, and between their world cities, in avoidable mortality than in total mortality. This lends support to the hypothesis that at least some of the difference between these countries can be attributed to differences in their health systems. The comparisons of the United States and Manhattan with England and London are also revealing. Our analysis shows that the health of residents of Inner London, measured in terms of total mortality and avoidable mortality, is worse than the health of Manhattan residents. Given the great concentration of deprivation in Inner London and its long-standing reputation for poor primary care (Evandrou, 2006), these results are not surprising.

We did not expect to find higher rates of avoidable mortality in England than in the United States unless all deaths due to IHD were excluded. Thus, while the NHS appears to have reduced the rates of many causes of avoidable mortality, our findings are consistent with concerns that the NHS may provide less access to effective specialty services, particularly those aimed at preventing and treating heart disease. To address health inequalities and improve access to primary care, the NHS created primary care trusts (PCT) in 2004. All general practitioners contracting with the NHS are now assigned to PCTs, which are charged with commissioning and providing health care, as well as monitoring the quality of care (Evandrou, 2006). In view of recent NHS reforms, our concerns that this analysis is based on only two short time periods, the lack of strictly comparable income data, and the major role of IHD in accounting for differences in avoidable mortality, we cannot conclude that the NHS has failed. Rather, our evidence suggests strong grounds to monitor rates of avoidable mortality in England and Inner London to evaluate the impact of recent NHS reforms.

It is troubling that, although Manhattan has lower rates of avoidable mortality than Inner London (even if deaths from IHD are excluded), inequality of access to timely and effective health care is a much greater problem in Manhattan than in either Paris or Inner London. The lower avoidable mortality rates in Paris suggest that geographic equity among rates of avoidable mortality across the city need not be the higher overall rates we observe in Inner London.

In contrast to Paris and Inner London, where there is universal health care coverage, in Manhattan those living in the poorest neighborhoods exhibit a significantly higher percentage of avoidable deaths than people living in the rest of the borough. Whether this is related to barriers in access to health care services, inadequate knowledge of the system's operation, or a lesser ability to communicate with providers is unclear. Perhaps, as suggested in the analysis of infant mortality (Chapter 2), this reflects patterns of racial segregation and other forms of discrimination that might affect both the incomes and access to health care of minorities in Manhattan. These differences in avoidable mortality may also relate to lifestyle choices, the probability of disease detection, and patient adherence to medical instructions, all of which have been related to socioeconomic status (Cavelaars, Kunst, and Mackenbach,1997; Lynch, Kaplan, and Salonen, 1997).

The leading causes of avoidable mortality in all three nations and urban cores suggest that disparities in access to screening services and to primary and specialty health care may explain the observed differences in rates. Further research is needed to improve our understanding of these disparities. All three cities have placed great emphasis, since the early 1990s, on primary and secondary prevention efforts, but we cannot assess the degree to which these efforts contributed to the observed decline in the rate of avoidable mortality. Although avoidable mortality is related more closely to the performance of the health system than are broader measures of health status, this correlation has limitations. The changes we observe between the two time periods may be due to broader social determinants of health—factors that are not reflected in avoidable mortality rates. They may also be explained by changes in the populations of these cities. For example, during the 1990s, the population of Manhattan became younger, wealthier, and better educated (Tobier, 2006). Comparable changes occurred in Inner London (Warnes, 2006). It is plausible, therefore, that some portion of the improvements in avoidable mortality may be due to such demographic change. On the other hand, the age distribution of the Paris population did not change significantly during this time, yet it experienced a 16 percent decline in the rate of avoidable mortality.

Summary

Avoidable mortality is an indicator that captures premature deaths due to conditions for which there are effective public health and health care interventions. Some components of avoidable mortality, such as maternal death, can be eliminated almost completely. In fact, dramatic reductions in maternal deaths, which are due primarily to direct obstetrical complications, are one of the greatest accomplishments of health care systems in the developed world during the last century. Furthermore, the failure to reduce these deaths in developing countries is one of the greatest sources of global health inequalities (Rosenfield, Min, and Freedman, 2007). Although most causes of premature death in the definition of avoidable mortality cannot be eliminated, even in wealthy countries, it is possible to reduce them significantly. High rates of avoidable mortality in a neighborhood or city suggest that residents of that area are not receiving life-saving health care services.

The comparisons in this chapter of rates of avoidable mortality across and within our three world cities and their respective nations highlight some of the stark differences among these cities, with regard not only to the aggregate performance of the three health systems but also in terms of geographic inequalities within them.

Inner London and England had the highest rates of avoidable mortality, while Paris and France had the lowest. Despite these differences, the rates declined in all three cities and countries during the 1990s. The decline in avoidable mortality was greatest in Manhattan, where the rate fell about 20 percent during this period. Regardless of this progress,

Manhattan's poorest residents have a significantly higher rate of avoidable mortality than other residents of the city. This suggests that barriers to access are greatest in the poor neighborhoods of Manhattan, but mortality data do not allow a precise identification of the factors that explain these differences.

For a more precise understanding of health care inequalities within these three cities, we analyze access to primary care and specialty services. In the next chapter, we examine a measure of health care access more closely related to primary care services: "avoidable hospital conditions." This measure captures the management of chronic diseases, such as congestive heart failure, asthma, and diabetes, which account for a significant number of hospitalizations in these countries. Indeed, because greater population longevity has been accompanied by a growth in chronic disease, it is important to understand how well these systems are coping with this challenge.

CHAPTER FOUR

Access to Primary Care

Avoidable Hospital Conditions

A VOIDABLE MORTALITY is a useful summary measure of health system performance, reflecting a range of health care interventions, from
primary and secondary prevention to tertiary care. Its breadth is both a
strength and weakness. An exclusive focus on avoidable deaths, however,
does not identify the contributions of public health, primary health care,
or specialty medical services. In this chapter, we refine our analysis of
access to care by comparing hospital discharge rates for avoidable hospital conditions (AHCs) across and within the three cities. AHCs are
inpatient hospitalizations for a host of conditions that, in theory, can be
"avoided" through timely access to effective primary health care. These
include hospitalizations for bacterial pneumonia, cellulitis, and several
chronic conditions, such as congestive heart failure, asthma, and diabetes. It is not possible to eliminate all hospitalizations for most of these
conditions, but access to primary care for their effective management
should significantly reduce the number of acute episodes leading to
hospitalization.

AHC is widely accepted as a valid measure of access to primary care. In
its 1993 report *Access to Health Care in America* (Millman, 1993), the
Institute of Medicine recommended that AHC rates be used to monitor
access to health care services at the national level and that these rates be
tracked over time to determine whether conditions for obtaining care
were improving or deteriorating, especially for vulnerable populations.
Since then, the Agency for Healthcare Research and Quality (AHRQ) has
used AHCs to monitor access to safety net services across large metropolitan areas of the nation (Billings, 2004), and the Commonwealth Fund is
publishing annual state-wide comparisons based on Medicare data (Cantor
et al., 2007).

Because many of these hospitalizations are for chronic conditions, comparing AHC rates also provides important information about how well health care systems are coping with the growing challenge of chronic disease (Ettelt et al., 2006; Olshansky et al., 2005). As the populations in these cities grow older, an increasing number of adults have multiple chronic conditions. If their care is not well coordinated, such adults are at risk for avoidable hospitalizations and other adverse events (Davis, 2007). To provide a broader context for our comparison of AHCs across and within our three cities, we begin with some background on the management of chronic disease and the challenge of comparing primary care systems.

Managing Chronic Disease

Four chronic diseases—cancer, cardiovascular disease, diabetes, and chronic lung diseases—are responsible for at least half of all deaths in the world each year (Suhrcke et al., 2006). Other estimates suggest that "more than four-fifths of all deaths and two-fifths of all disabilities" can be attributed to these four diseases—and nearly half of these deaths are premature (Stuckler, 2008: 276). One estimate in the United States suggests that the care of chronic disease accounts for 78 percent of national health expenditures (Anderson and Horvath, 2002). Over the past decade, the incidence of diabetes worldwide has nearly doubled (International Diabetes Federation, 2006). Current projections suggest that by 2020, one-tenth of the world's population will have diabetes (Suhrcke et al., 2006). Increases in diabetes and other chronic diseases threaten to curb the gains in longevity achieved over the past 30 years, not to mention quality of life (Olshansky et al., 2005), and contribute to rising health care costs (Thorpe and Howard, 2006). Moreover, the growth of chronic disease is most relevant for the study of health systems in world cities because globalization and urbanization are often cited as factors contributing to its growth (Stuckler, 2008).

Because the care of people with chronic conditions accounts for a disproportionate share of health expenditures, policy makers across the world are struggling to improve coordination of health services for patients with chronic conditions. For example, interest in disease management and primary care gatekeeping has grown in Europe since the late

1990s. In 2004, France enacted a health care reform plan under the leadership of health minister Philippe Douste-Blazy. The most important feature of the law was to promote the development and application of managed care techniques, including computerized medical records, practice guidelines, and incentives to encourage primary care physicians to coordinate health services for their patients. At present, more than 85 percent of the French population has signed up with a *médecin traitant* (primary care physician). Moreover, one of the key architects of the health care reform plan, Fréderic Van Roekeghem, director general of the union of national health insurance funds (Union Nationale des Caisses d'Assurance Maladie, or UNCAM), has promoted disease management techniques.

In the United Kingdom, the national service frameworks of Department of Health and Social Security (DHSS) have promoted strategies to reduce hospitalizations for various conditions. In 2000, the department issued a national service framework for the treatment of coronary heart disease and the following year for diabetes. The national service framework for chronic conditions was published in 2005. These frameworks are part of a larger effort to address health disparities and improve the performance of primary care doctors. They set national standards, define service models, develop strategies to support implementation, and establish performance measures against which progress is measured. As in the case of France, the impact of these reforms is not yet clear and requires careful monitoring.

Along with establishing national service frameworks, the NHS and DHSS have funded a host of additional projects designed to improve coordination of health care services for people with chronic conditions. For example, between 2002 and 2004 the DHSS funded and supported a community-based pilot program for each primary care trust (PCT) to provide training for people in the self-management of long-term conditions. Nearly all of the 300 PCTs in England participated, and almost 10,000 people enrolled in the program. Among participants, there was a 7 percent reduction in general practitioner consultations, a 10 percent reduction in outpatient visits, a 16 percent reduction in accident and emergency room visits, and a 9 percent reduction in the use of physiotherapy. In addition, some PCTs are adopting so-called pay-for-performance incentives into their contracts with general practitioners. In the Torbay Primary Care Trust, for example, general practitioners can earn £100 for every patient with chronic illness whom they keep out of the hospital.

Comparative Analysis of Primary Care Systems

A common problem in comparative studies of health care systems is the lack of common terminology. Cross-national comparisons of primary care illustrate this well. The term *primary care* has different meanings in different countries; the failure to define the term carefully inhibits the ability of researchers and policy makers to learn from each other (Mullan, 1998). In some nations, primary care is any health care delivered by general practitioners. In other countries, *primary care* refers to a specific set of services, regardless of who delivers it. In a reflection of these differences, Ettelt and colleagues found that the range of services that primary care physicians provide varies across countries. In England and other national health service systems, general practitioners provide a comprehensive set of services, but in France and other national health insurance systems, "patients are more likely to seek specialist services for first-contact care" (Ettelt et al., 2006: 7). There are many reasons for these differences, including the availability and political power of specialists as well as differences in medical education and tradition (Ettelt et al., 2006; Mullan, 1998).

In many countries, the idea that primary care is a mechanism for controlling resources is popular. As Mullan explains, "The concepts of risk management, disease management, and demand management are receiving attention in highly regulated medical sectors such as Germany's, just as they are in the U.S. market-driven environment. These ideas inevitably lead to the concept of a clinical manager who will be responsible in some fashion for decisions about medical care and, therefore, resource use" (Mullan, 1998: 125).

Along with the lack of cross-national agreement regarding the definition of primary care—and perhaps because of it—we have little comparative information about how primary care is organized among different health care systems. The literature that compares health systems documents the number of physicians and hospital beds in different countries, but "there is surprisingly little information currently available about how different countries deliver care outside hospitals" (Ettelt et al., 2006: 2). This information gap is striking because there is a widespread belief that primary care is an important component of all health systems. Starfield and colleagues, for example, argue that a good system of primary care can and should (1) mediate the effects of other health determinants;

(2) improve preventive care and reduce preventable deaths; (3) reduce the ill health effects of social inequalities associated with income and resource distribution; and (4) improve overall referral, coordination, and continuity of care in a health system (Casanova and Starfield, 1995; Macinko, Starfield, and Shi, 2003; Shi et al., 1999; Shi and Starfield, 2000). Similarly, researchers from the Commonwealth Fund claim that greater reliance on primary care is one of the distinguishing characteristics of "high-performing" health systems (Schoen, Davis, et al., 2006).

In addition to controlling resources, there is some evidence that systems with primary care gatekeepers provide continuity and integration of care (Ettelt et al., 2006; Macinko, Starfield, and Shi, 2003; Shi et al., 1999; Shi and Starfield, 2000). The indicators of health system performance established by the OECD Health Promotion Prevention and Primary Care Panel are based, in part, on the premise that "the coordination of care among different providers and the provision of guidance to patients through the health care system are key functions of primary health care" (Marshall et al., 2004: 8). Among our three cities, there have been efforts to use primary care as a "gatekeeper" in Manhattan and Inner London, but in Paris—and the rest of France, as we noted earlier—the implementation of what might be termed *soft gatekeeping* is relatively new.

Whether or not primary care doctors are asked to serve as gatekeepers in the system, Starfield and colleagues marshaled evidence, mostly from the United States, that systems with more primary care providers achieve better health outcomes (Starfield, Shi, and Macinko, 2005). Studies using a variety of methods, and controlling for a number of other factors such as age, education, ethnicity, income, and race, have concluded that the density of primary care physicians is associated with better health outcomes (Starfield et al., 2005). The supply of primary care providers is associated with higher life expectancy at birth and lower infant mortality (Vogel and Ackerman, 1998), lower mortality from all causes (Shi et al., 2003), lower disease-specific mortality (Campbell et al., 2003), and higher self-reported health status (Shi and Starfield, 2000). Other studies find that the ratio of primary care providers to specialists is associated with better outcomes (Gusmano, Rodwin, and Cantor, 2006; Shi, 1992, 1994). Although it is possible that the association between the supply of primary care and these outcomes is not causal, there is strong circumstantial evidence that primary care improves the performance of a health system.

We focus here on one important dimension of primary care: the management of illnesses and chronic conditions to reduce avoidable hospitalizations. This approach is useful for several reasons.

First, examining the consequences of poor access to timely and effective primary care allows for the possibility that there may be more than one way to manage these illnesses effectively, so this approach does not require an a priori determination of the institutional arrangements necessary for a "good" primary care system. The use of a primary care gatekeeper is often presumed to be a necessary element of a successful primary care system. Because of the heavy weighting they place on this dimension of primary care, Macinko and colleagues claim that France has one of the worst systems of primary care among OECD nations. Using 1995 data, they ranked France below the United States, Germany, and Switzerland (Macinko, Starfield, and Shi, 2003). Their ranking system uses a 0- to 2-point scale for each of 10 dimensions.* France received zeroes on several of the dimensions, including not requiring first contact with a primary care provider; failing to use guidelines for the transfer of information between primary care providers and other levels; failing to regulate the distribution of primary care providers; requiring "cost sharing" for primary care visits; not having comprehensive services available at primary care sites; failing to organize patient records by "family" rather than by individual; and failing to use community-based data in primary care.

Despite this dismal assessment of the French primary care system, we find that rates of AHCs are lower in Paris than in Manhattan and Inner London and that disparities among neighborhoods in Paris are lower, as well.† Our finding does not negate the importance of the factors identified by Macinko and colleagues, but it does raise important questions about the validity of such criteria for assessing the performance of primary care systems. It is possible that Paris has a low rate of AHCs *in spite of* its primary care system, but this conclusion would, among other things, force us to reject a large body of evidence that supports the validity of AHCs as a measure of access to timely and effective primary

---

* The 10 dimensions are regulation, financing, dominant type of primary care provider, access, longitudinality, first contact, comprehensiveness, coordination, being family-centered, and being community-centered.

† We also found that the rate of AHCs is significantly lower for France than for England, Germany, and the United States (Gusmano, 2008).

care. It seems more likely that the Macinko assessment tool is incomplete, or perhaps too narrowly focused on institutional arrangements that may promote the coordination of care but that are not necessary to achieve it.

The second reason for focusing on the management of illnesses and chronic conditions is that we can measure this dimension of primary care using definitions and data sources that are comparable across these systems. Finally, as we discuss below, chronic disease is a growing concern for all health care systems, so better understanding of how these three cities are addressing the problem may provide useful insights for other cities and nations trying to cope with similar challenges. In all three urban cores, there is a concentration of primary care physicians and clinics. Even in Manhattan, where residents face greater financial barriers and primary care physicians represent a smaller proportion of the total physician workforce than in Paris or Inner London, residents have access to one of the largest health care safety nets in the world, composed of public hospitals, community health centers, and other primary care clinics. The question is whether the existence of this health care safety net is sufficient to meet the growing primary care needs of the population in the context of a health care system where there are severe gaps in health insurance coverage.

Are Avoidable Hospital Conditions Valid Indicators of Access to Primary Care?

In discussions about how health systems can ensure access through a combination of health insurance coverage, availability of primary care doctors, and safety net providers, AHCs are recognized in the literature in the United States, Canada, Spain, and Britain as valid indicators of access to primary care (Brown, Goldacre, and Hicks, 2001; Casanova and Starfield, 1995; Sanderson and Dixon, 2000).* Although some studies question whether AHCs can reliably distinguish health system characteristics from the socioeconomic status of their populations (Blustein, Hanson, and Shea, 1998), there is widespread agreement that differences in AHC rates among neighborhoods reflect disparities in access to primary

---

* AHCs are also known as "ambulatory care sensitive conditions" (ASCs).

care, not population health status (Ansari, 2007; Oster and Bindman, 2003; Wennberg, 1987).

Some of the conditions that are included in the definition of an AHC are completely avoidable through immunization. For example, we should not see any hospitalizations for polio. Other hospitalizations can be avoided if the condition is caught early and managed well. For many of the conditions included in our definition of AHCs, it is not likely that any health system would be able to eliminate all hospitalizations. Yet, if these conditions are managed effectively, it should be possible to reduce significantly the number of acute episodes that result in hospitalizations.

How many hospitalizations could be avoided? This is difficult to estimate precisely, but the total hospitalizations due to AHCs in the countries we examine are enormous, and the potential savings associated with reducing such hospitalizations, even by a modest amount, are great. In France, which has the lowest rate of AHCs among the countries we examine, there are more than 400,000 hospitalizations for AHCs among adults each year. In England, there are more than 600,000 hospitalizations for AHCs among adults each year.

Is it reasonable to expect the United States to reduce its rate of AHCs to the same level as France or England? Perhaps not, but before we can assess this possibility, we must first identify the features of these systems that help to explain the differences among them. To that end, we analyze AHCs in Manhattan, Inner London, and Paris.

Studies in the United States have found that the uninsured are more likely to be admitted to hospitals with AHCs because they are less likely to receive effective and timely primary care than those with insurance (Billings, Anderson, and Newman, 1996; Pappas et al., 1997; Parchman and Culler, 1994). Differences in disease prevalence, not in access to care, may explain the differences in hospital discharge rates for AHCs among areas of low and high socioeconomic status (Blustein, Hanson, and Shea, 1998). Given the findings of the relevant literature, however, we are confident that the prevalence or severity of disease in a population does not explain the differences in hospital discharge rates for AHCs for two reasons.

First, a number of previous studies suggest that the prevalence or severity of disease in the population is unlikely to explain the differences in hospital discharge rates for AHCs (Billings et al., 1993; Casanova and Starfield, 1995; Weissman, Gatsonis, and Epstein, 1992). For example,

Weissman and colleagues controlled for baseline hospital use, race, and income, which they argue should correct for differences in need or demand for hospital services (Weissman, Gatsonis, and Epstein, 1992: 2393). They concluded that access to primary care, which was particularly poor among the uninsured, and not differences in health status, explained the differences they observed.

Second, comparison of hospital discharge rates for AHCs with so-called marker conditions enables one to distinguish access issues from those related to disease prevalence. Unlike discharge rates for AHCs, hospital discharge rates for "marker conditions" are not influenced by access to ambulatory care. These are conditions for which previous use of ambulatory care does not affect the risk of hospitalization. They do not vary greatly by socioeconomic status or neighborhood of residence, and the extent to which they vary is more likely an indicator of differences in morbidity or other measures of population health status. What we expected to see with the marker conditions was no difference among geographic areas. For example, one of the marker conditions is appendicitis, which would not be prevented even if a person had received high-quality primary care in the months, or years, before being hospitalized for this condition. Moreover, rates of hospital discharge due to appendicitis and other marker conditions tend to fall within a narrow band. Billings and colleagues include hospitalizations due to heart attacks in the definition of marker conditions (Billings, Anderson, and Newman, 1996). We exclude this diagnosis from our definition because, although access to timely and effective primary care during the weeks immediately before a heart attack is unlikely to prevent the heart attack, there may be a role for primary care in reducing the risk of developing coronary artery disease in the months or years before hospitalization. Therefore, to ensure that we are including only causes of hospitalization that have little, if anything, to do with access to primary care, we limit our definition of marker conditions to appendicitis, gastrointestinal obstruction, and hip fracture.

Hypotheses, Measures, and Data Sources

Previous research has examined hospitalization rates for AHCs and marker conditions in major urban areas of the United States. Our study is the first such comparison of Manhattan, Inner London, and Paris.

Because of our findings on avoidable mortality (Chapter 3), we expected that AHC rates would be highest among residents of Manhattan and lowest among Parisians. Although we found that the rate of avoidable mortality was highest in Inner London, we suspect that this pattern is driven by deaths due to IHD and several forms of cancer. The high avoidable mortality rate in Inner London could be the result of poor access to primary care, but we suspect it is driven more by access to specialty care, surgery, and pharmaceuticals.

Because residents of Manhattan and London are less healthy than residents of Paris, we also expected that hospital discharge rates for marker conditions would be higher in Manhattan and London, though not as great as the differences among AHC rates. If disparities among rates of AHCs reflect only differences in the use of hospitals as a site of care, we would expect higher rates of AHCs in Paris than in Manhattan because the total hospitalization rate is higher in Paris.

For a measure of income, we used pretax, median household income by neighborhood in Manhattan and Paris and the deprivation index in London. For the logistic regressions, we calculated neighborhood income quartiles on the basis of currencies in Manhattan (U.S. dollars) and Paris (euros) and on the deprivation index for Inner London.

To calculate hospital discharge rates for AHCs, we used the definition of an AHC developed by Joel Weissman and colleagues (1992), which has been validated by previous studies (Backus et al., 2002; Pappas et al., 1997; Parchman and Culler, 1994). The Weissman definition includes pneumonia, congestive heart failure, asthma, cellulitis, perforated or bleeding ulcer, pyelonephritis, diabetes with ketoacidosis or coma, ruptured appendix, malignant hypertension, hypokalemia, immunizable conditions, and gangrene.

To calculate rates for marker conditions, we calculated hospital discharge rates for appendicitis without abscess or generalized peritonitis, gastrointestinal obstruction, and hip fractures (Billings, Anderson, and Newman, 1996). (For more information about the hospital administrative data used in this analysis, see the Appendix.)

We calculated hospital discharge rates of AHC, marker conditions for age-adjusted cohorts, employing the direct standardization method and using the 2000 United States standard population to obtain adjustment weights (Klein and Schoenborn, 2001). We calculated age-adjusted rates for each city for above- and below-median income neighborhoods and used difference of means tests to examine the statistical significance of the differences. To assure an adequate number of hospital discharges and procedures for statistically meaningful comparisons, and to reduce the likelihood that an annual anomaly might affect the results, we calculated averages over a four-year period (1998–2001) for each city (Fig. 4.1).

We found that for persons 18 years or older, the age-adjusted rate of AHCs in Manhattan (16.1 per 1000) is more than 50 percent higher than that of Paris (6.9) and 40 percent higher than the rate in Inner London. These differences are much greater than the differences found among large U.S. cities, which have AHC rates comparable to Manhattan's (Billings and Weinick, 2003). In contrast, discharge rates for marker conditions are only about 11 percent higher in Manhattan than in Inner London, and Manhattan and Paris are nearly identical. That marker condition rates are so similar suggests that differences among the cities with regard to rates of AHCs are due to differences in access to care, not merely a reflection of differences in population health status or the role of acute care hospitals.

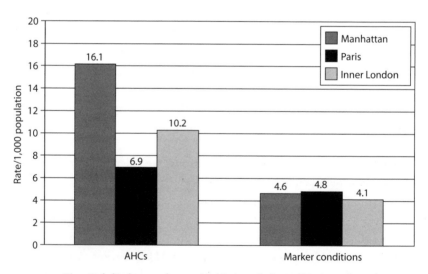

FIG. 4.1. Hospital discharges for avoidable hospital conditions and marker conditions, Manhattan, Paris, and Inner London: age-adjusted rates for persons 18 and older, 1998–2001 averages.

What Factors Influence Rates of Avoidable Hospital Conditions?

People without health insurance in the United States are less likely to have a usual source of care, use physician services, or undergo elective tests and procedures, and are more likely to delay or forego care than their insured counterparts (Aday et al., 1998; Berk, Schur, and Cantor, 1995; Brown, Wyn, and Teleki, 2000; Kasper, Giovannini, and Hoffman, 2000; Saver, 1996; Weissman, Gatsonis, and Epstein, 1992). As noted earlier, the uninsured also have disproportionately high rates of hospital admissions for conditions that are believed to be directly linked to deficiencies in access to primary, preventive care (Billings, Anderson, and Newman, 1996; Hadley, Steinberg, and Feder, 1991; Weissman et al., 1992).

Yet, while many studies suggest a correlation between avoidable hospitalizations and insurance status, most fail to disentangle the relative importance of insurance coverage, other barriers to access, poverty, and education (Blustein, Hanson, and Shea, 1998). Blustein and colleagues found, for example, that differences in "preventable hospitalizations" among Medicare beneficiaries were due primarily to low socioeconomic status rather than access to primary care. All three cities studied here have neighborhoods with high concentrations of poverty and low levels of education. In Manhattan and Inner London, in particular, persons living in lower-income neighborhoods report that they are less likely to have a usual source of care (Rodwin and Gusmano, 2006a). As a result, it is reasonable to think that AHC rates may be elevated in lower-income areas within all three cities—but we expected to find that these differences are much greater in Manhattan, which has the highest levels of material inequality and the largest neighborhood health disparities.

In an effort to disentangle the factors that explain differences across and within these cities, we present results from multiple logistic regression models in Tables 4.1–4.3. These models estimate the effects of both individual and neighborhood characteristics on the probability of hospitalization for AHCs in each city. We ran separate regression equations, rather than pooling the hospital data, and we included a dummy variable for each city because we do not have identical co-variates for each city. The French hospital administrative database, Programme de Médicalisation

TABLE 4.1. Manhattan: logistic regression results for characteristics associated with admission for avoidable hospital conditions (dependent variable) for persons age 18 and above

Independent variable	Coefficient (S.E.)	P > |z|	% change in odds for unit increase in X
Age (continuous)	0.0231 (0.0003)	0.000	2.3
Female (omitted = male)	−0.1244 (0.0015)	0.000	−0.12
Race/ethnicity (omitted = white)			
Black	0.2528 (0.0144)	0.000	29
Hispanic	0.3275 (0.0144)	0.000	47
Other race	0.1147 (0.0139)	0.000	12
Income quartile of zip code (omitted = highest)			
Lowest	0.3605 (0.0205)	0.000	43
Second	0.2437 (0.0186)	0.000	27
Third	0.1384 (0.0163)	0.000	15
Number of diagnoses on record (continuous)	0.0231 (0.0003)	0.000	2.4
Insurance status (omitted = private insurance)			
Medicare	0.1884 (0.0154)	0.000	21
Medicaid	0.3275 (0.0149)	0.000	39
Uninsured	0.5963 (0.0210)	0.000	82
Other government programs (Champus, prison, etc.)	0.3327 (0.0210)	0.000	38
Physicians/1,000 for zip code population	−0.0015 (0.00078)	0.0460	−0.01

des Systèmes d'Information (PMSI), does not include information about payer, or race or ethnicity.

For all three cities, our models estimate the probability that an individual is hospitalized with an AHC. For Manhattan, the independent variables are age, gender, race/ethnicity, number of diagnoses on the record

TABLE 4.2. Paris: logistic regression results for characteristics associated with admission for avoidable hospital conditions (dependent variable) for persons age 18 and above

Independent variable	Coefficient (S.E.)	P > |z|	% change in odds for unit increase in X
Age (continuous)	0.0169 (0.0003)	0.000	1.7
Female (omitted = male)	−0.3562 (0.0104)	0.000	−30
Income quartile of arrondissement (omitted = highest)			
Lowest	0.0243 (0.0244)	0.320	2.5
Second	0.0229 (0.0188)	0.226	2.3
Third	−0.0091 (0.0184)	0.621	−1
Arrondissement with > 40% adult population without a baccalaureate degree	0.02759 (0.0157)	0.079	2.8
Number of diagnoses on record (continuous)	0.0829 (0.0018)	0.000	8.6
Physicians/1,000 for arrondissement population	−0.0118 (0.0028)	0.000	−1.2

(as a measure of severity of illness), and primary payers (Table 4.1). The model also controls for a number of the neighborhood variables at the zip code level: income quartile, physician density, and dummy variables for zip codes in which more than 15 percent of the households are linguistically isolated and more than 40 percent of the adult population do not have a high school diploma.*

In Paris, the independent variables are age, gender, and number of diagnoses; the neighborhood variables for arrondissements are indicators for income quartile, physician density, and an education dummy variable for arrondissements in which more than 40 percent of the adult population

* We ran a model with secondary payers and interactive terms relating race and zip code, income and race, and insurance. These variables did not change the results, so we dropped them from the final model (see the Appendix), and they are not shown in Table 4.1.

TABLE 4.3. Inner London: logistic regression results for characteristics associated with admission for avoidable hospital conditions (dependent variable) for persons age 18 and above

Independent variable	Coefficient (S.E.)	$P > |z|$	% change in odds for unit increase in X
Age (continuous)	0.022	0.000	2.3
Female (omitted = male)	−0.247	0.000	−21.9
Race/ethnicity (omitted = white)			
Black	−0.100	0.000	−9.6
Asian	0.038	0.050	3.8
Other	−0.009	0.280	−1
Deprivation quartile of borough of residence (omitted = highest)			
Most deprived	0.070	0.001	7.3
Second most deprived	−0.013	0.414	−1.1
Third most deprived	−0.032	0.0020	−1.3
Number of diagnoses on record (continuous)	0.075	0.000	7.8
Percentage of borough population reporting poor health	−0.001	0.001	−1
Physicians/1,000 for borough population	0.016	0.000	1.6

do not have a baccalaureate degree (Table 4.2). (The French baccalaureate degree is the equivalent of completing high school and a first year of college in the United States.) The Paris model does not include race/ethnicity or linguistic isolation because the French census does not include such indicators. Nor does the model have a measure for payer source because the French hospital administrative database does not include this information. Although the French national health insurance system includes multiple payers, the benefit packages and reimbursement levels are virtually identical, so there is no meaningful difference among them.

In Inner London, the independent variables are age, gender, race/ethnicity, and number of diagnoses on the record (as a measure of severity of illness) (Table 4.3). The model also controls for a number of the neighborhood variables at the borough level: deprivation quartile, percentage of the population reporting poor health, and physician density.

Because the observations about individuals from the same neighborhood may be correlated, we tested for bias due to unobserved neighborhood-level heterogeneity by estimating the models with a dummy variable for each zip code or arrondissement as a replacement for neighborhood-level variables. The estimates for the individual characteristics were not appreciably different from those generated by these models. (See the Appendix.)

In Manhattan, women have much lower odds of admission for AHCs (12%). There are also small but statistically significant influences for increasing age, number of diagnoses, and physician density (Table 4.1). The relationships among zip code of residence median household income, race, and insurance status on AHCs in Manhattan, however, are statistically significant and large. The odds of AHCs are about 29 percent higher among African Americans and 47 percent higher among Hispanics than among whites. The odds of AHCs for persons without health insurance are about 82 percent greater than for persons with private insurance. The odds are 39 percent higher among Medicaid recipients and 21 percent higher among Medicare beneficiaries than among persons who have private health insurance. The odds of AHCs are about 43 percent higher among residents of the poorest neighborhoods, 27 percent higher among residents of the second poorest neighborhoods, and 15 percent higher among residents of the third poorest neighborhoods, compared with the wealthiest neighborhoods of Manhattan.

The odds ratios calculated for Paris reveal a statistically significant, but very small, influence for age, number of diagnoses on the record, and physician density. As we found in Manhattan, the odds of admission for AHCs are lower among women than among men. Indeed, the gender difference was much greater in Paris, where the odds are about 30 percent lower for women than for men. The neighborhood income and education variables are not significant in Paris (Table 4.2).

Our findings for Inner London are remarkably similar to those for Paris (Table 4.3). In Inner London, age, place of residence, physician density, and the percentage of people in the borough who report being in poor health do not much influence the odds of being hospitalized for an AHC. The odds of being hospitalized for an AHC are almost 10 percent lower for blacks than for whites, and there is little difference between whites and Asians or other ethnic groups. The only factor we examined that seems to matter a great deal is gender. As in Paris and Manhattan, the odds of being hospitalized with an AHC are much lower for women (22%) than for men.

Limitations of Analysis and Alternative Explanations

We are unable to account directly for any effect of differences in disease prevalence on rates of AHCs, but previous research suggests that this factor is unlikely to explain the differences we observed. For example, Oster and Bindman (2003) argue that higher rates of AHCs among African Americans and Medicaid patients do "not appear to be explained by either the differences in disease prevalence or disease severity." Similarly, Laditka and colleagues (2003) find that higher rates of AHCs among African Americans and Hispanics, compared with non-Hispanic whites, are not due to differences in disease prevalence. The notion that underlying prevalence of disease is unlikely to explain differences in rates of AHCs is reinforced by the work of Wennberg (1987), who finds that population illness rates do not explain hospitalization rates.

The race and insurance effects we observed in Manhattan and the gender effects noted for both cities may be the result of patients' compliance or care-seeking behavior. It is also possible that the behavior of physicians may influence these rates (Weissman, Gatsonis, and Epstein, 1992). Despite this concern, others suggest that physician practice style is unlikely to explain the differences we observe (Komaromy et al., 1996). Our data do not permit us to test these alternative hypotheses.*

Summary

In all three urban cores, AHC rates are correlated with neighborhood-level income. Although this association is evident, the disparity between high- and low-income neighborhoods is greatest in Manhattan. As noted in Chapter 3, there is much greater race-based residential segregation and geographic concentration of poverty among blacks and other ethnic minorities in all U.S. cities, including Manhattan, than in European cities. Our comparison of geographic disparities in the rate of AHCs supports

---

* Although our use of dummy variables is an accepted technique when both individual and group-level variables are included in the same model, we plan to refine this analysis by using multilevel modeling in future work on Manhattan and Inner London. It is impossible to run a multilevel model for Paris using the French hospital reporting system, PMSI, because there are not enough observations for the level-2 (group) variables to create a hierarchical linear model.

the claim that an important consequence of Manhattan's concentration of poverty in particular neighborhoods results in greater disparities in access to health care.

Women have much lower odds of being admitted to a hospital for AHCs in these cities. This is consistent with well-known gender differences in the use of ambulatory care—it is higher among women than men (Muller, 1990)—but the similarity of the gender difference across these urban cores is remarkable given the large differences in the total rates of AHCs. It suggests that none of these systems is doing a particularly good job of encouraging men to make use of primary and preventive care.

Despite these similarities, Manhattan stands out in comparison with Inner London and Paris. While age-adjusted discharge rates for marker conditions are only slightly higher, the age-adjusted rate of AHCs in Manhattan is more than 60 percent higher than in Inner London and about 250 percent higher than in Paris. The difference between Manhattan and Paris is remarkable because the aggregate hospital discharge rate is higher in Paris. Our findings therefore provide strong evidence that the health care systems in Paris and Inner London perform better in terms of admitting to hospitals a far lower share of patients for AHCs.

These findings are consistent with other studies and suggest that the higher rates of AHCs in Manhattan are explained by multiple barriers to care, including race and ethnicity, income, gender, and insurance status. Medicare beneficiaries, Medicaid recipients, and the uninsured are all more likely to be hospitalized for AHCs than are individuals with private health insurance. African Americans and Hispanics are also more likely to be hospitalized for AHCs than non-Hispanic whites.

Our comparison of Manhattan, Paris, and Inner London documents some important consequences of access barriers in a city that is known for its strong health care safety net institutions. In Manhattan, the magnitude of AHCs is considerably higher than in Inner London and Paris, where all residents benefit from universal coverage in health systems that have effectively eliminated financial barriers to health care. Although our findings suggest that insurance is only one of several barriers to care in Manhattan, it is clearly important. Often, we assume in the United States that the existence of public hospitals, community health centers, and other safety net institutions enable the uninsured to obtain the care they need (Brown, 2003). An important implication of this analysis is that we should not devote disproportionate attention to strengthening the health care safety net at the expense of extending health insurance coverage (Cunningham and Hadley, 2004).

Inadequate health insurance coverage in the United States contributes to a lack of timely, effective primary care. This often results in unnecessary illness, loss of productivity, and costly, preventable hospitalizations. It is difficult to quantify the magnitude of unnecessary illness and loss of productivity, but the total hospitalizations due to AHCs in the countries we examined are enormous, and the potential savings associated with reducing such hospitalizations, even by a modest amount, are great. In France, which has the lowest rate of AHCs of the three countries, there are more than 400,000 hospitalizations for AHCs among adults each year. In England such hospitalizations exceed 600,000, and in the United States there are more than 2.5 million.

CHAPTER FIVE

Access to Specialty Care

The Treatment of Heart Disease

Despite a recent decline in its incidence, ischemic heart disease (IHD) remains the world's leading cause of death as well as a major contributor to health care expenditures. France has a much lower IHD mortality rate than most other nations belonging to the Organization for Economic Cooperation and Development (OECD). Indeed, the IHD mortality rate in France is less than half that of the United States and England. The low IHD mortality rate in France, coupled with the country's reputation for consuming large quantities of high-fat foods, is a phenomenon often dubbed the "French paradox" (Renaud and Gueguen, 1998).

Cross-national comparisons indicate that the United States provides higher rates of cardiac catheterization and revascularization procedures—percutaneous transluminal coronary angioplasty (PTCA) and coronary artery bypass graft (CABG) surgery—than France and other OECD nations (Moise and Jacobzone, 2003). A study based on the most recent state-of-the-art international comparison of the use of high-tech interventions concludes that the United States is more aggressive than Canada, Scotland, Sweden, Israel, Australia, and Denmark in providing procedures following heart attacks (Technological Change in Health Care Research Network, 2001). The English National Health Service (NHS) is well known for its low rates of revascularization, particularly among older people (Aaron, Schwartz, and Cox, 2005).

This chapter compares the use of revascularization in our three nations and urban cores. When we examined age-adjusted rates of revascularization without attempting to account for national and city-level differences in the burden of coronary heart disease, our findings were consistent with those we have noted, but when we adjusted for the burden of disease in these three nations and their world cities, the contrast between our findings and those of previous comparisons were striking. At the national level, the ratio of revascularization to acute myocardial infarction (AMI) among persons 65 years or older is highest for residents of France. Although this ratio is lowest among residents of England for all age groups, the differences we found are much smaller than previous studies suggest.

When we accounted for the burden of disease in our urban cores, we found that Parisians receive revascularizations at a higher rate than residents of Manhattan for all age groups. We believe this is largely because the rate of revascularization in Manhattan among racial and ethnic minorities and the uninsured is so low. The rate of revascularization is lowest among residents of Inner London and is particularly low among residents of the most deprived boroughs in the city and ethnic minorities, but the difference is smaller than the differences found by Aaron, Schwartz, and Cox (2005), which are based on national data alone.

Another remarkable finding is the similar gender disparity in the use of revascularization procedures in these urban cores. Gender disparity in the treatment of heart disease has been a concern in the United States for some time, but most population-based studies ignore this issue, and there have been few efforts to extend this analysis beyond the United States. We found that, in all three urban cores, use of these procedures is significantly lower among women (Weisz, Gusmano, and Rodwin, 2004). Indeed, despite significant differences among these cities with regard to the use of revascularization, the magnitude of the gender disparities we found was almost identical. Even after we accounted for differences in disease, women receive 27–28 percent fewer revascularizations than men in all three cities.

The Reliability of Comparisons of Heart Disease and Its Treatment across Nations

Comparing rates of disease and surgery among nations is a challenge because of differences in coding and interpretation of data. For our comparison, we took care to avoid some of the common mistakes associated with cross-national comparisons of revascularization.

We obtained U.S. data for hospital discharges and rates of PTCA and CABG from the National Hospital Discharge Survey, National Center for Health Statistics. As with our analysis of avoidable hospital conditions (Chapter 4), we obtained these data for Manhattan, by area of residence, from the Statewide Planning and Resource Cooperative System (SPARCS) and for both France and Paris from the French Ministry of Health's hospital administrative database, Programme de Médicalisation des Systèmes d'Information (PMSI).* For England and London, we obtained Hospital Episode Statistics (HES) data on patients treated in the NHS from the Department of Health and Social Security. As in Chapters 3 and 4, to ensure an adequate number of hospital discharges, procedures, and deaths for meaningful comparisons, we calculated 4-year averages (1998–2001).

Information on coronary revascularization funded by private payments is not routinely collected in the United Kingdom and must be obtained by surveys. The estimated private contribution varies from 7 to 30 percent (Black et al., 1996; Williams et al., 2000). The most recent estimates for London, based on a review of data gathered from every private hospital in London, suggest that including privately funded revascularizations would increase the figure in HES by about 15 percent (Mindell et al., 2008). In terms of the relative position of our nations and cities with regard to the use of revascularization, the exclusion of these private revascularizations does not matter: even if we increase the estimates for England or Inner London by 30 percent, they still provide far fewer procedures than the other countries and cities. However, using the number of privately funded revascularizations does reduce the disparity between England and other OECD nations.

The WHO MONICA Project (Multinational Monitoring of Trends and Determinants of Cardiovascular Disease) highlights some of the difficulties associated with comparing death rates across populations (Tunstall-Pedoe et al., 1994). For example, project investigators observed that documentation of nonfatal cardiac events was more reliable than mortality, in part because a large proportion of deaths were unclassifiable due to a lack of diagnostic information or any medical history. When categorizing nonfatal episodes, they classified events as definite events, possible events, or "no myocardial infarctions" using only ECG criteria because cardiac enzyme criteria are neither universally available nor

* As noted in Chapter 4, PMSI centralizes discharge data from all French hospitals by diagnosis, procedure, age, and current address of patients. All hospitals with more than 100 beds provide data to this system. The exclusion of hospitals with fewer than 100 beds presents no problem for the analysis of revascularization because these procedures are not performed in smaller hospitals.

standardized (Burke, Edlavitch, and Crow, 1989). National IHD mortality rates are clearly not uniform within countries in the MONICA study, and as noted earlier, mortality data may not be reliable.

Some researchers have expressed concern that the differences in criteria for ascribing death to IHD in France may be the reason for the lower French rates (Artaud-Wild et al., 1993; Nestle, 1994; Renaud and Gueguen, 1998). To address these concerns, we relied on hospital discharge data to test the reliability of the mortality data. These hospital discharge data can validate findings where accepted clinical diagnostic criteria exist, as in the case of acute myocardial infarction (AMI). Other national comparisons focus on broad categories of coronary artery disease or IHD, but these categories include conditions for which diagnoses are less reliable, such as congestive heart failure (CHF) (Akosah et al., 2001). To avoid omitting patients who might have been misdiagnosed or miscoded, we adopted a conservative strategy and identified patients using the International Classification of Diseases-9-CM and ICD-10 diagnostic codes for AMI, as well as all IHD. Examining AMI separately acts as a check on the reliability of broader categories.

Our use of SPARCS, HES, and PMSI data on procedure rates for residents of Manhattan, London, and Paris avoids a common misinterpretation of the number of CABG procedures in the United States. OECD estimates are based on a sample of inpatient records from short-stay hospitals in the United States (National Hospital Discharge Survey, National Center for Health Statistics), which are widely disseminated in the Heart and Stroke Statistical Update of the American Heart Association. The data for cardiac revascularization (bypass: ICD-9 codes 36.1–36.3) are presented as procedures (553,000 in 1998) and as patients (336,000 in 1998). The "procedure" variable represents the number of coded procedures recorded, but for a given operative procedure on a single patient either a single code (representing an arterial or a venous conduit bypass) or two codes (employed when a combination of arterial and venous conduits have been used) may be counted. The frequent use of two codes for what is in fact a single operative procedure exaggerates the number of procedures performed in the United States by about 61 percent (OECD, 2001).

To analyze differences in invasive treatment for IHD, we calculated age-adjusted rates of revascularization (PTCA and CABG) for two cohorts: 45–65 years and 65 years or older. We did not examine diagnostic cardiac catheterization or coronary angiography rates because they are often performed as outpatient procedures in all three countries and cities. As a result, data on their volume, particularly at the level of the urban core, are unreliable.

The Relationship between Treatment Rates and the Burden of Disease

To assess the relationship between treatment rates and the burden of IHD, we used a simple index based on the ratio of procedure rates to AMI mortality rates. Although the true burden of IHD in any population will never be known because the illness may be asymptomatic, we examined both mortality and hospital discharge rates for AMI as a proxy for the burden of IHD. We do not intend to suggest that every person who has an AMI receives one of these procedures. Nor do we suggest that this is the only diagnosis for which these procedures are an appropriate intervention. Our examination of the ratio of procedure rates to AMI mortality rates is merely an attempt to adjust for the different burden of heart disease among our nations and cities.

In 2000, both the European Society of Cardiology and the American College of Cardiology recommended changing the diagnostic criteria for AMI to include raised troponin T concentrations in addition to changes in electrocardiograms. The use of this new diagnostic tool may increase the number of people diagnosed with AMI, but this change is unlikely to affect our results, for three reasons. First, our data are from 1998 to 2001, so the 4-year averages would not be influenced significantly by these new recommendations. Second, there is no evidence that the examination of troponin T concentrations is more prevalent in one of these nations or cities than in the other two. Third, we conducted a sensitivity analysis in which we substituted other measures of heart disease burden (hospitalizations for all IHD, hospitalizations for AMI, and mortality due to all IHD) in the denominator of our index. The results did not change greatly when we used these alternative measures of heart disease. While our index represents a preliminary effort limited by available data, failure to consider some measure of disease burden when analyzing treatment rates is clearly misleading (OECD, 2006; Technological Change in Health Care Research Network, 2001).

What Do We Know about the Burden of Heart Disease in World Cities?

Mortality rates due to AMI and IHD in Manhattan and Paris reflect the well-known differences in mortality from heart disease between the United States and France. Manhattan residents exhibit higher mortality rates than their Parisian counterparts for AMI and all IHD. This contrast is more pronounced with age. For those 65 years or older, rates of mortality due to AMI in Manhattan are 60 percent higher than in Paris; for those age 45–64, they are 35 percent higher.

Curiously, mortality rates due to all IHD are slightly lower in England than in the United States for both age cohorts, and they are lower in Inner London than Manhattan among persons 65 and older. The mortality rate due to AMI is highest in England and Inner London: while it is nearly identical to the rate in the United States among persons 45–64, it is 24 percent higher among persons 65 and older. The problem is even more pronounced in Inner London, particularly among adults 45–64 years old, for whom the mortality rate due to AMI is 104 percent higher than in Manhattan. Among older persons, the mortality rate due to AMI is 30 percent higher in Inner London than in Manhattan, a percentage comparable to the national-level difference (Table 5.1).

U.S. and Manhattan residents exhibit a higher rate of hospitalization for AMI and ischemic heart disease than residents of France and Paris (Table 5.2). Once again, the contrast is more pronounced for older persons than for those between the ages of 45 and 64. For those 65 years and over, hospital discharge rates due to AMI in Manhattan are 49 percent higher; for people 45–64, they are only 29 percent higher. Thus, when we compare the United States and Manhattan with France and Paris, the comparison of hospital admission rates is consistent with the differences in mortality rates.

The hospital discharge comparison with England and Inner London is less consistent with the mortality comparison. Even though mortality rates due to AMI are higher in England than in the United States for both age cohorts, hospital discharge rates due to AMI are more than 40 percent lower. By contrast, when we compare Inner London with Manhattan, the hospital discharge rates due to AMI are higher in Inner London among persons 45–64 and only about 8 percent lower among persons 65 and older.

TABLE 5.1. Age-adjusted mortality rates for acute myocardial infarction (AMI) and all ischemic heart disease (IHD), 1998–2001

	45–64 age cohort		65+ age cohort	
	Rate/ 100,000[a] (N)	% difference from Manhattan/ U.S.[b]	Rate/ 100,000[a] (N)	% difference from Manhattan/ U.S.[b]
	AMI (ICD-9 = 410)			
Manhattan	23.5 (83)		372.0 (716)	
Paris	15.3 (77)	−35.0	150.1 (556)	−59.6
Inner London	48.0 (240)	103.9	482.4 (1,346)	29.7
United States	52.7 (32,525)		460.3 (161,001)	
France	27.9 (3,838)	−47.1	212.2 (21,125)	−53.9
England	55.6 (7,324)	0.1	571.3 (47,349)	24.1
	AMI IHD (ICD-9 = 410–414)			
Manhattan	83.3 (295)		1,377.8 (2,661)	
Paris	22.2 (112)	−73.3	320.1 (1,213)	−76.8
Inner London	131.7 (660)	58.0	1,187.1 (3,317)	−13.8
United States	110.7 (68,344)		1,194.8 (417,916)	
France	37.3 (5,141)	−66.3	391.2 (39,355)	−67.3
England	103.88 (13,671)	−6.1	1,143.3 (94,732)	−4.3

DATA SOURCES: Manhattan—Office of Vital Statistics, New York City Department of Health; United States—Centers for Disease Control and Prevention, National Vital Statistics Report; France and Paris—Institut National de la Santé et de la Recherche Médicale (INSERM); England and Inner London—Department of Health and Social Security.

[a] Average rates over 4-year period.

[b] Percentage difference from Manhattan for cities and from the United States for countries.

TABLE 5.2. Residence-based hospital discharge rates for acute myocardial infarction (AMI) and all ischemic heart disease (IHD), 1997–2001

	45–64 age cohort		65+ age cohort	
	Rate/ *100,000*[a] *(N)*	*% difference* *from* *Manhattan/* *U.S.*[b]	*Rate/* *100,000*[a] *(N)*	*% difference* *from* *Manhattan/* *U.S.*[b]
	AMI (ICD-9 = 410)			
Manhattan	166.2 (585)		692.6 (1,303)	
Paris	117 (587)	−29.6	322.9 (1,113)	−53.4
Inner London	219.5 (1,089)	32.1	637.7 (1,800)	−7.9
United States	430.2 (254,600)		1,427.2 (490,600)	
France	256.2 (35,036)	−38.4	730.3 (71,117)	−48.8
England	249.7 (32,251)	−42	837 (69,500)	−41.4
	All IHD (ICD-9 = 410–414)			
Manhattan	676.9 (2,389)		2,168.4 (4,044)	
Paris	607.6 (3,053)	−10.2	1,485.1 (4,832)	−31.5
Inner London	1,072.2 (5,323)	58.4	2,549.3 (7,240)	17.6
United States	1,332.6 (788,400)		3,652.2 (1,255,200)	
France	841.8 (115,113)	−36.8	2,065 (199,884)	−43.5
England	907.6 (117,453)	−31.9	2,344.4 (194,819)	−35.8

DATA SOURCES: Manhattan—Statewide Planning and Research Cooperative System (SPARCS); United States—National Hospital Discharge Survey; France and Paris—French Ministry of Health's Hospital Reporting System (Programme pour la Médicalisation des Systèmes d'Information, PMSI); England and Inner London—Hospital Episode Statistics (HES).

[a] Average rates over 4-year period.

[b] Percentage difference from Manhattan for cities and from the United States for countries.

We see a similar pattern when we examine hospital discharge rates due to IHD. The rates are more than 30 percent lower in England than in the United States, but they are 59 percent higher in Inner London than in Manhattan among persons 45–64 and 18 percent higher in Inner London than in Manhattan among persons 65 or older.

The Use of Revascularization

When we examine age-adjusted rates of revascularization without attempting to account for national- and city-level differences in disease rates, our findings are consistent with previously reported national findings. The age-adjusted rate of revascularization is highest in the United States. The differences in the age-adjusted rates of revascularization among the urban cores are consistent with the national figures but not nearly as pronounced.

One problem with the data on revascularization among residents of England and Inner London is that, although the HES database includes revascularizations conducted in private hospitals but paid for by the NHS, it does not include data on hospitalizations or procedures that are conducted in private hospitals and financed with private funds—either out-of-pocket payments or private health insurance. If we use the recent estimate of Mindell and associates (2008), which suggests that about 15 percent of revascularizations for Londoners are funded privately, the rate for England moves closer to the rate in France (and other countries in Europe), and that for Inner London moves closer to the rates of its world city counterparts (Table 5.3).

When we use our index to adjust for the burden of disease in the three nations and cities, the contrast between our city-level findings and those of previous cross-national comparisons is striking. The ratio of revascularization procedure rates to AMI mortality rates is only 2 percent higher in the United States than in France among persons 45–64, and it is 5 percent *lower* in the United States than in France among persons 65 years or older. The comparison between the United States and England does not change substantially when we examine our ratio: the ratio of revascularization procedures to AMI mortality rates is 75 percent lower in England among persons 45–64 and 87 percent lower among persons 65 years or older. Given the high AMI mortality rate in England, this is not surprising.

TABLE 5.3. Rates for age-adjusted revascularization procedures, 1998–2001

	45–64 age cohort		65+ age cohort	
	Rate/ 100,000[a] (N)	% difference from Manhattan/ U.S.[b]	Rate/ 100,000[a] (N)	% difference from Manhattan/ U.S.[b]
Manhattan	309.7 (1,093)		893.7 (1,655)	
Paris	257.3 (1,293)	−16.9	525.8 (1,653)	−41.2
Inner London	227.3 (1,131)	−26.6	365.5 (1,049)	−59.1
United States	630.2 (373,200)		1,342.2 (461,400)	
France	327.4 (44,773)	−48.0	648.4 (62,185)	−51.7
England	167.6 (21,747)	−73.4	223.5 (18,633)	−83.3

DATA SOURCES: Manhattan—Statewide Planning and Research Cooperative System (SPARCS); United States—National Hospital Discharge Survey; France and Paris—French Ministry of Health's Hospital Reporting System (Programme pour la Médicalisation des Systèmes d'Information, PMSI): England and Inner London—Hospital Episode Statistics (HES).

[a] Average rates over 4-year period.
[b] Percentage difference from Manhattan for cities and from the United States for countries.

The ratio of revascularization procedure rates to AMI mortality rates is substantially higher in Paris than in Manhattan for both age cohorts. The ratio is lowest in Inner London for both cohorts, but the difference between Inner London and the other urban cores is not as great as the difference between England and the other nations (Table 5.4).

What explains the lower use of revascularization procedures in the United States compared with France among older adults, and in Manhattan compared with Paris among *all* adults? One possibility is that residents of France, and to a greater extent, those of Paris, receive too many of these procedures as a result of physician-induced demand made possible by universal coverage, coupled with minimal access barriers to care (Lucas-Gabrielli, Pépin, and Tonnellier, 2006). Another possibility is that residents of the United States, and to a greater extent, Manhattan, face stronger

TABLE 5.4. Ratio of rate of age-adjusted revascularization to rate of age-adjusted mortality from acute myocardial infarction (AMI), 1998–2001

	45–64 age cohort		65+ age cohort	
	Ratio of revasculariza- tion to AMI	% difference from Manhattan/ U.S.[a]	Ratio of revasculariza- tion to AMI	% difference from Manhattan/ U.S.[a]
Manhattan	13.18		2.40	
Paris	16.82	22	3.50	31
Inner London	4.74	–64	0.76	–68
United States	11.96		2.92	
France	11.73	–2	3.06	5
England	3.01	–75	0.39	–87

DATA SOURCES: Manhattan—Statewide Planning and Research Cooperative System (SPARCS); United States—National Hospital Discharge Survey; France and Paris—French Ministry of Health's Hospital Reporting System (Programme pour la Médicalisation des Systèmes d'Information, PMSI); England and Inner London—Hospital Episode Statistics (HES).

NOTE: We use mortality rates for AMI as a proxy for estimated disease prevalence. The index we calculate for assessing the use of these procedures is the result of dividing age-adjusted procedure rates for the population residing in each geographic area, irrespective of where the procedures were performed, by the age-adjusted rates of mortality from AMI. Thus, higher indices reflect higher levels of service in relation to our proxy for estimated disease prevalence. For additional discussion of this indicator, see the Appendix.

[a] Percentage difference from Manhattan for cities and from the United States for countries.

access barriers to specialty care than do their French counterparts and therefore do not receive needed procedures. Our data do not allow us to comment on appropriateness of care, but previous studies suggest that large geographic variations in the United States can be attributed to factors other than disease burden (Pilote et al., 1995). These have included age (Pashos, Newhouse, and McNeil, 1993), race (Ayanian et al., 1993), sex (Ayanian and Epstein, 1991; Leape et al., 1999), income, co-morbid conditions, location of care, and health insurance status (Carlisle, Leake, and Shapiro, 1997; Philbin et al., 2001). Other studies point to an inverse relationship between distance to health care personnel or facilities and use of services (Ben-Shlomo and Chaturvedi, 1995; Blustein, 1993; Gregory et al., 2000; Grumbach, 1995). We conducted logistic regression analyses to investigate the extent to which each of these factors is correlated to rates of revascularization for residents 45 years or older of Inner London, Manhattan, and Paris hospitalized with IHD or congestive heart failure.

Intracity Disparities in Access to Revascularization within World Cities

In keeping with our overall approach to world city comparisons, it is not sufficient to compare differences among our cities if we want to understand how these urban health systems influence access to health care services. It is also important to examine disparities in access to care within these cities. Thus, we present results from multiple logistic regression models, which estimate the probability that a person hospitalized with IHD or congestive heart failure will receive a revascularization procedure (PTCA or CABG).

For Manhattan, the independent individual variables are age, gender, race/ethnicity, primary payers, and number of diagnoses on record (as a measure of severity of illness); the neighborhood variables, at the zip code level, are indicators for income quartile and physician density (Anderson, 1995). We also ran a full model with secondary payers, as well as interactive terms relating race and zip code income, and race and insurance. These interactive terms and secondary insurance variables did not change the results, so we dropped them from the final model.

For Paris, the independent individual variables are age, gender, and number of diagnoses on record (as a measure of severity of illness); the neighborhood variables, at the arrondissement level, are indicators for income quartile and physician density. For Inner London, the independent individual variables are age, gender, race/ethnicity, and number of diagnoses on record; the neighborhood variables, at the borough level, are indicators for deprivation and physician density.

We include the variable "age squared" in all three models, in addition to continuous age variables, because the probability of revascularization increases between the ages of 45 and 75 but decreases thereafter due to increasing frailty. Because the observations on individuals from the same neighborhood may be correlated, we tested for bias due to unobserved neighborhood-level heterogeneity by estimating the models with a dummy variable for each zip code as a replacement for neighborhood-level variables. The estimates for individual characteristics were not appreciably different from those generated by the original model (Greene, 2000).

In Manhattan, we find that insurance status, race, gender, zip code of residence, and number of diagnoses are all related significantly to the probability of revascularization among residents of Manhattan diagnosed with IHD. Residents of the lowest-income zip codes are significantly less likely to receive revascularization than residents of the highest-income areas. In Manhattan, the odds of being hospitalized with IHD and receiving revascularization are 28 percent lower among women than among men (Table 5.5).

The odds of revascularization among those hospitalized with IHD are 48 percent lower among African Americans and 21 percent lower among Hispanics than whites. In contrast, the odds are 44 percent higher among Asians and others than whites, but given the small number of persons in this category hospitalized for IHD, this result requires further investigation.

The odds of revascularization are 62 percent lower for persons without health insurance than for persons with private insurance. The odds are 65 percent lower among Medicaid recipients, and 31 percent lower among Medicare beneficiaries, than among persons with private health insurance. The odds of revascularization are about 61 percent lower for persons with "other" government health insurance, but much like the "other" race/ethnicity category, these results may be due to small numbers.

To illustrate further the influence of insurance status on access to revascularization, we used the New York City Community Health Survey (New York City, 2004a) to estimate a population denominator for the persons with private insurance, Medicare, Medicaid, other insurance, and no insurance in Manhattan. Doing so allowed us to calculate our ratio of age-adjusted revascularizations rates to age-adjusted AMI mortality rates separately for each group in Manhattan. The ratio for persons with private health insurance is identical to the ratio for all residents of Paris. As the regression analysis suggests, it is substantially lower for all of the other groups, particularly people who are uninsured.

In Paris, the continuous age variable is positively correlated with revascularization, but when we examine age squared, there is a small but statistically significant relationship. The density of physicians is not related

TABLE 5.5. Manhattan: Logistic regression results for characteristics associated with revascularization for persons age 45 and above hospitalized with heart disease

Independent variable	B (S.E.)	% change in odds for unit increase in X
Age (continuous)	0.22860***	25.7
	(0.002)	
Age squared	−0.00196***	−0.2
	(.001)	
Female (omitted = male)	−0.32999***	−28.1
	(.027)	
Race/ethnicity (omitted = white)		
Black	−0.65699***	−48.2
	(.047)	
Hispanic	−0.23957***	−21.3
	(.042)	
Asian and "other"	0.36151***	43.5
	(.032)	
Income quartile zip code (omitted = highest)		
Lowest	−0.42428***	−34.6
	(.031)	
Second	−0.29820***	−25.8
	(.041)	
Third	−0.24675***	−21.9
	(.036)	
Number of diagnoses on record (continuous)	−0.02902***	−2.9
	(.004)	
Insurance status (omitted = private insurance)		
Medicare	−0.37020***	−30.9
	(.036)	
Medicaid	−1.05268***	−65.1
	(.044)	
Uninsured	−0.97806***	−62.4
	(.075)	
Other government insurance	−0.94664***	−61.2
	(.711)	
Physicians/1,000 for zip code population	0.00062	0.1
	(.001)	

*** .001 level of significance
No. of observations = 48,306

significantly to revascularization. Although we find that persons with more diagnoses on their record and people with a higher severity score are less likely to receive a revascularization, neither has a large effect on the odds of revascularization (Table 5.6).

The influence of gender and neighborhood income on the odds of revascularization in Paris are, however, both significant and large. The odds of revascularization are 21 percent lower among residents of the lowest-income arrondissements compared with residents of the highest-income arrondissements. Similarly, the odds of revascularization are 23 percent lower among residents of the second-lowest-income arrondissements and 14 percent lower among the third-lowest compared with the highest-income arrondissements. As we discuss below, women are far less likely to receive revascularization than men (Weisz, Gusmano, and Rodwin, 2004).

TABLE 5.6.   Paris: logistic regression results for characteristics associated with revascularization for persons age 45 and above hospitalized with heart disease

Independent variable	B (S.E.)	% change in odds for unit increase in X
Age (continuous)	0.21219***	23.6
	(0.01)	
Age squared	−0.00180***	−0.2
	(0.00)	
Female (omitted = male)	−0.30742***	−26.5
	(0.04)	
Income quartile of arrondissement (omitted = highest)		
Lowest	−0.23402***	−20.9
	(0.07)	
Second	−0.26620***	−23.4
	(0.05)	
Third	−0.14643***	−13.6
	(0.05)	
Number of diagnoses on record (continuous)	−0.05419***	−5.3
	(0.01)	
French IGS-2 index of severity for Paris (continuous)	−0.00549*	−0.5
	(0.00)	
Physicians/1,000 for arrondissement population	0.00176	0.2
	(0.01)	

* .05 level of significance
*** .001 level of significance
No. of observations = 31,359

Unlike our findings on avoidable mortality and avoidable hospital conditions for Inner London (Chaps. 3 and 4), there are substantial racial, gender, and geographic disparities in access to revascularization within this urban core. Not only do residents of Inner London receive fewer revascularizations than do residents of the other two cities, but also the disparities we observe within Inner London are comparable to those that exist in Manhattan (Table 5.7). We find that race, gender, borough of residence, and number of diagnoses are all related significantly to the probability of revascularization among residents of Inner London diagnosed with IHD.

TABLE 5.7. Inner London: logistic regression results for characteristics associated with revascularization for persons age 45 and above hospitalized with heart disease

Independent variable	B (S.E.)	% change in odds for unit increase in X
Age (continuous)	0.338	40.2
	(0.014)	
Age squared	−0.003	−0.1
	(0.000)	
Female (omitted = male)	−0.321	−27.4
	(0.025)	
Race/ethnicity (omitted = white)		
Black	−0.309	−26.6
	(0.058)	
Asian	0.041	4.2
	(0.043)	
Other	−0.153	−14.1
	(90.026)	
Income-related quartile of borough (omitted = highest)		
Most deprived	−0.765	−53.5
	(0.065)	
Second most deprived	−0.010	−0.1
	(0.045)	
Third most deprived	−0.043	−4.2
	(0.038)	
Number of diagnoses on record (continuous)	−0.118	−11.1
	(0.007)	
GPs/1,000 for quartile ward population	0.025	2.6
	(0.007)	

The odds that a resident of one of Inner London's most deprived boroughs will receive a revascularization are more than 53 percent lower than the odds for a resident of one of the least deprived boroughs. Curiously, however, the odds of revascularization among residents of boroughs in the second and third income quartiles are not very different from the odds for residents living in Inner London's least deprived boroughs. The HES database does not include patients who receive privately financed revascularizations, but the analysis by Mindell and colleagues (2008) suggests that the inclusion of these patients would increase the geographic disparities we observe in Inner London. Patients who purchase and use private health insurance for such procedures are more likely to receive them and more likely to live in the city's least deprived boroughs.

As we found in the other urban cores, the odds that women hospitalized with IHD will receive revascularization in Inner London are lower (27%) than for men (Table 5.7). In addition to these factors, we examined the role of ethnicity in Inner London. The odds of revascularization among those hospitalized with IHD are 27 percent lower among blacks,* and about 14 percent lower among "other" non-Asian ethnic minority groups, than among whites. In contrast, the odds are 4 percent higher among Asians than whites. These findings are consistent with a host of recent studies that highlight the problem of ethnic disparities within the NHS (Evandrou, 2006; National Health Service and Commission for Racial Equality, 2004).

Gender Disparities in Treatment of Heart Disease

Not only did our effort to account for differences in disease burden allow us to compare geographic and other disparities within these cities and nations more effectively than previous studies, but it also allowed us to explore gender disparities in the treatment of heart disease within and among these places. While this issue has received considerable attention in the United States, it has not been explored abroad. Our findings suggest that gender disparities in the treatment of heart disease are a common phenomenon in each of our three nations and their world cities. To assure

---

* Black African and Black Caribbean combined.

meaningful numbers, and because women tend to experience the onset of heart disease 6–10 years later than men, we focus on treatment of men and women 65 years and older.

The impression that heart disease is a "man's disease" and not an urgent concern in women has resulted in treatment patterns that appear to give short shrift to women with heart disease. Even when heart disease is recognized as a problem in women, it is generally associated with the "older old" (75+) and is often not well documented or properly investigated. Between 1979 and 1998, the rate of mortality attributed to AMI decreased much more rapidly in men 65 years and older than in women in the same age group.*

Our analysis points to significant gender disparities in the incidence of procedures for IHD. The consistency of our results across nations and cities is striking given the differences in treatment rates for IHD. Despite disparities in the use of CABG and PTCA that reflect differences in health system characteristics, there is a consistent pattern of gender disparity in the treatment of IHD.

Although the gender gap in the incidence of IHD has been explored in the literature (Barrett-Connor, 1997), the reasons for the disparity remain unclear. Women with AMI are twice as likely to die from the event as men, at least in part because of the occurrence of AMI at an older age and in those with more co-morbid conditions (Tunstall-Pedoe, 1988). Nonetheless, there is no evidence to support the significantly lower rates of revascularization for women which we observed (Williams et al., 2000).

The discrepancy between the sexes may be the result of sociocultural or biological factors. For example, there were differences in the clinical profiles, presentations, and outcomes in men and women with acute coronary syndromes in the Global Use of Strategies to Open Occluded Coronary Arteries in Acute Coronary Syndromes angioplasty substudy (GUSTO IIb) that could not be accounted for by differences in baseline characteristics (Hochman et al., 1999). Although the investigators concluded that the findings could be explained by variations in underlying anatomy or pathophysiology, they also observed gender differences in the rates of referral for diagnostic testing and revascularization. This finding raises the possibility of a gender bias.

* As documented by the CDC (www.cdc.gov/nchs).

Studies from Boston (Steingart et al., 1991) and Chicago (Bergelson and Tommaso, 1995) reported lower rates of diagnostic coronary angiography in women that were related to age and the interpretation of symptoms. However, having undergone catheterization, women were found to be as likely to undergo angioplasty as men but less likely to undergo CABG, based on both age and gender (Healy, 1991). A study from the United Kingdom reported similar findings in patients with a diagnosis of AMI or IHD. There was no gender difference in the use of revascularization overall, but men were more likely to undergo CABG (Raine et al., 2002).

Whether being a woman is an independent risk factor for a poor outcome after surgical revascularization remains controversial. Whereas some data indicate that female gender is no longer a predictor of increased risk (Golino et al., 1991; Mickleborough et al., 1995), particularly after adjustment for body size (O'Connor et al., 1993), other studies have concluded that gender is a risk factor (Khan et al., 1990). Similarly, although earlier studies of PTCA reported poorer results in women (Bell et al., 1993; Cowley et al., 1985), a more recent study described better outcomes for women than men (Jacobs et al., 1998).

Data collected for administrative purposes may be used to analyze patterns of clinical care, as we have done here. Yet these data, which typically contain only limited information on patient demographic characteristics, discharge diagnoses, and procedure codes, make it impossible to adjust adequately for risk factors and differences in disease severity or comorbidities. The results of some clinically based studies suggest that certain gender differences disappear after controlling for various risk factors, whereas other studies do not support this suggestion (Bickel et al., 1992; Rahimtoola et al., 1993; Vaccarino, 2002). A more clinically detailed data set might explain our findings concerning gender differences; however, even a study that directly examined gender differences in the severity of illness provided no explanation because use of different severity measures produced different estimates of whether women were sicker than men (Iezonni et al., 1997).

A multiplicity of intangible and subjective factors influence medical decision-making: the doctor-patient relationship, unconscious physician bias (Sheifer, Escarce, and Schulman, 2000), patient preference (and the extent to which it is influenced by age and gender) (Cleary, Mechanic, and

Greenley, 1982; Saha, Stettin, and Redberg, 1999), and, not least, practice patterns—whether related to professional "uncertainty" (Wennberg, Barnes, and Zubkoff, 1982) or "enthusiasm" (Chassin, 1993). Although our data do not allow us to assess the magnitude of the role played by these factors, our findings highlight the importance of conducting such assessments. In addition, our data did not allow us to assess the appropriateness of the procedures studied (i.e., whether they were "overused" in men or "underused" in women). Rather, our findings highlight the need for additional research to evaluate these and other influences on the observed gender disparities.

The magnitude of the gender disparities observed in the treatment of IHD in Manhattan, Inner London, and Paris is clear. The odds that women will receive a revascularization are more than 25 percent lower than men in all three cities. Moreover, despite differences in populations, health systems, health insurance coverage, medical resources, and medical culture, this pattern was consistent. The existing literature indicates that the observed disparities cannot be explained on the basis of either clinical data or patient preferences.

These findings call for more clinical and population-based research to examine the extent to which gender disparities result in inappropriate use of advanced medical procedures. Such analyses will require detailed data on individual-level socioeconomic and clinical variables. The present evidence is sufficient to support development of policies to encourage increased physician awareness of gender disparities and thus improve the care of women with IHD.

Summary

Our findings regarding hospital discharge rates by area of patient residence, for AMI as well as IHD, are consistent with previous cross-national comparisons of heart disease in France and the United States. Death rates are higher in the United States and Manhattan, as well as England and Inner London, than in France and Paris. Likewise, hospital discharge rates for AMI and all IHD provide strong evidence that the burden of IHD is significantly higher in the United States and Manhattan, and England and Inner London, than in France and Paris (Table 5.2). Moreover, the disparity in disease burden between the United States and France and

Manhattan and Paris increases with age, and mortality rates from all IHD are about three times as high in the United States and Manhattan as in France and Paris.

A recent comparison of trends in invasive procedures for patients with heart disease indicates that the United States provides higher rates of cardiac catheterization, PTCA, and bypass surgery within one year of a heart attack than do the other high-income OECD nations in the study (Technological Change in Health Care Research Network, 2001). Similarly, a comparison of the United States and Canada in the GUSTO-1 study found that the rates of PTCA and CABG following AMI among Canadian patients were much lower than any of the regional rates reported for the United States (Rouleau et al., 1993).

Our analysis of revascularization rates in the United States, France, England, and Manhattan, Paris, and Inner London differs markedly from that in the literature on cross-national comparisons. Once we account for the higher disease burden in the United States, it appears that older residents of France receive more revascularization procedures than their American counterparts. Residents of England receive far fewer revascularizations, but the difference is not as dramatic as some previous estimates, particularly once we account for privately funded revascularizations. In London, the inclusion of privately funded revascularizations increases the total by about 15 percent, but we do not know what this figure would be for the entire country.

At the city level—where our analysis is in many respects more refined because these cities are more similar than their countries in terms of sociodemographic characteristics and medical resources—we find that Manhattan residents receive invasive procedures at a significantly lower rate than Parisians. The use of revascularization is much lower among residents of Inner London than in Manhattan or Paris, but the differences are not as great as they are at the national level. Our observation that residents of Inner London receive far more revascularizations than do residents of England is not surprising because although Inner London has fewer hospital beds and surgeons than its world city counterparts, the supply of medical resources is greater in Inner London than in the rest of the country.

Our logistic regression analysis indicates that women and residents of lower-income neighborhoods are less likely to receive revascularization procedures in all three cities. In Manhattan, the effect of neighborhood income is strongest. Insurance and race present additional barriers to residents of Manhattan. Despite the commitment of the NHS to allocate care on the basis of need, race is a significant barrier in Inner London as well (Propper and Upward, 1992).

It is possible that lower rates of revascularization in the low-income arrondissements of Paris reflect barriers that could be attributed to race and ethnicity as well. It is illegal to collect such data in France, so it is impossible for us to investigate this question.

Without patient-specific clinical data it is, of course, not possible to disentangle the role of these factors from strictly clinical criteria in explaining the use of cardiac procedures, but our findings are consistent with other studies that identify nonclinical barriers to high-tech treatment modalities in Manhattan and the United States (Ayanian and Epstein, 1991; Ayanian et al., 1993; Grumach et al., 1995; Philbin et al., 2001).

Our evidence cannot address issues related to the appropriateness of care for residents of these cities or nations. Indeed, it is possible that many of the people who receive these procedures do not benefit from them. Nevertheless, our findings underscore the possibility that many people who need these procedures fail to receive them because of nonclinical barriers to medical care. Such a finding illustrates the added value of supplementing cross-national studies with city-level comparisons. Although our analysis appears entirely consistent with the characterization of the U.S. health care system as one marked by "excess and deprivation" (Enthoven and Kronick, 1989), we present a different story from the one told by most of the cross-national health systems literature. Our analysis suggests that the United States provides more revascularizations than other developed nations, not primarily because U.S. hospitals and surgeons have an economic incentive to provide more of these procedures, but because their patients have more heart disease. Yet, the response to this greater need varies substantially by the race, gender, and the insurance status of the patient—contributing to the high rates of avoidable mortality we noted in Chapter 3, and leading to substantial welfare losses (Glied and Little, 2003).

CHAPTER SIX

Conclusions

THE THREE CITIES we compare in this book are among a small set of unique urban environments, with populations that are uncommonly large, diverse, and mobile. These world cities are also exceptionally well endowed with health care resources, innovative public health systems, sophisticated urban infrastructures, and financial markets that attract capital from around the world. Despite the density of their health care resources, however, they have shocking—some would say embarrassing—health inequalities. Disparities in population health, as well as access to primary and specialty care services, are most glaring in New York City.

New York City's public health system is well known for the size of its workforce, the extent of its programs, and the innovative nature of its disease surveillance capacities. The overall management of critical public health functions is more integrated at the local level than in Paris or London, where many public health functions are managed by separate agencies of the central state. In New York City, the U.S. federal government and New York State allow the city's Department of Health and Mental Hygiene to exercise greater autonomy over its public health programs than in Paris or London. After decades of neglect following New York's fiscal crisis in the 1970s (Socolar et al., 2001), the city has strengthened its public health infrastructure, its capacity for surveillance, and its efforts to reduce health disparities. Our findings, however, point to key limitations in New York City's capacity to address the health needs of its population. The enormous disparities in access to primary and specialty health services among residents of Manhattan, which we document in this book, reflect to a large extent a set of overlapping national policies in areas ranging from the economy to housing, the environment, education, and health care.

In our previous book, *Growing Older in World Cities*, we argued that "even the centralized unitary states of Japan, France and the United Kingdom have been unable to meet the needs of the oldest old without close collaboration of local government, nonprofit organizations, community and neighborhood organizations and families" (Gusmano and Rodwin, 2006a). The same can be said for the health and health care needs of city residents. People fall through the cracks of national policies and programs in all of these countries. All three of the cities we examine here work to fill these gaps—but the gap that must be filled by New York City government is significantly greater than that faced by the other cities. The growth in the number of uninsured and the large population of undocumented immigrants make this challenge even more daunting.

Why Is It Useful to Compare Health Systems in Cities?

Historically, the literature on cities and urban planning has largely ignored issues of public health and the organization of health services, while the literature on health services research has given the role of cities short shrift. From the heyday of nineteenth-century European public health movements, which focused on the importance of sanitation (clean water supply, sewers, and garbage disposal) and improvements in housing conditions, to twentieth-century interventions aimed at improving access to health services, the main body of research on public health, as well as on medical care, focused on cities. Moreover, the triumph of public health is largely responsible for making cities more habitable. Yet the field of urban studies has mostly ignored public health (Coburn, 2004), and the field of health services research has followed the growth of the welfare state in veering away from local territorial concerns and focusing on statistical aggregates ranging from regions, states, and nations.

The costs of segregating inquiry among the fields of urban planning and health services and policy research have been increasing with the growth of urbanization around the world because there is increasing awareness that the city is indeed a strategic unit of analysis for understanding the health sector. Yet most health services and policy research—both in the United States and among international organizations such as the United Nations, the World Health Organization (WHO), and the Organization for Economic Cooperation and Development (OECD)—continues to assume that states or nations as a whole are the most relevant units of analysis for assessing the performance of health systems and health policy. There are many limitations to this approach.

First, there are enormous variations in health and health system performance within nations, between urban and rural areas, between large and small cities, and between depressed and prosperous cities. Many studies of urban health have documented evidence of an urban health penalty for subpopulation groups living in cities (Andrulis and Shaw-Taylor, 1996; Geronimus, 1996). Other studies have focused on disparities in health status among different groups (New York City, 2004b). In addition, the Robert Wood Johnson Foundation's Tracking Project has highlighted disparities in resource levels and health system performance among midsize cities across the United States (Ginsberg, 1996).

Second, it is exceedingly difficult to disentangle the relative importance of health systems from other determinants of health, including the sociocultural characteristics and the neighborhood context of the population whose health is measured (Ellen, Mijanovich, and Dillman, 2001). It is even more difficult to do so at a level of aggregation such as the nation state where important dimensions of health policy are made.

Third, despite the rise of the welfare state, many health and social problems cannot be addressed by national and state governments even in the most centralized nations. Some of the most challenging problems—care for vulnerable older persons, people with severe mental illness, the most economically disadvantaged, and the uninsured—fall into a kind of residual category of problems that are passed down to local governments, among which city governments bear a disproportionate share (Rodwin and Gusmano, 2006a).

For all of these reasons, there is a good case for integrating inquiry across the fields of urban studies and health policy research. Among those concerned with cities, this will require a new focus on the health sector and measures of population health. Among those involved in health policy research, it will require special attention to health systems and population health in cities, which will, in turn, require disaggregated data on health services and health at the city and neighborhood levels.

Are World Cities Good for Your Health?

In a rapidly urbanizing world, New York, Paris, and London—in contrast to most megacities of the global South—have a recent history of relative success in assuring their population's health and share a range of characteristics and problems. They are great centers for prestigious teaching hospitals, medical schools, and medical research institutions. Despite these resources and the success of public health reformers and urban planners in improving their quality of life, these world cities still confront onerous health risks for at least four problems. The first of these is the return of infectious diseases (e.g., tuberculosis) and the emergence of new ones—AIDS, SARS, and influenza (H1N1). The second problem is terrorism, including bioterrorism, and emergencies stemming from climate changes (e.g., heat waves) (Cadot, Rodwin, and Spira, 2007). Since the release of toxic sarin gas in Tokyo's subway, bombs in the Paris and London subways, and the events of 9/11 followed by anthrax in New York and beyond, there has been an acute awareness of these risks. Third, there are the barriers in access to health care services for ethnic minorities and poor people. This has been recognized as a problem not just in New York City but also in Paris and London. Finally, cities face rising inequalities among social groups. This is reflected in the simultaneous growth of homelessness, poverty, and wealth in all three cities.

These problems will challenge any big city to develop a solid public health infrastructure. With or without such investments, there is already widespread belief that the health of urban populations is not as good as that of the population as a whole. This belief is supported by a substantial body of work, but those who disagree point to contrary evidence.

THE SICK CITY

Because the city is, by definition, the place where human density is greatest, it is hardly surprising that the city is a vector for the transmission of infectious disease. The Chicago Department of Health has collected data on basic measures of population health for 46 large cities across the United States, which have since been updated and published in the *Big City Health Inventory* (National Association of City and County Health Officials, 2007). Such measures (e.g., average incidence rates for infectious diseases like tuberculosis, AIDS, and syphilis) are much higher in these cities than for the United States as a whole. Also, these cities have much higher rates of mortality due to noncommunicable diseases (e.g., heart disease and cancer). Another important source on urban health in the United States, a compendium of data on the 100 largest cities (Andrulis and Shaw-Taylor, 1996), also reveals a greater prevalence of health problems in cities than in suburbs and rural areas, suggesting that there is an urban health penalty (Andrulis, 1997).

In Europe, a valuable source of information on urban health among capital cities comes from Project Mégapoles, which has compared age-specific mortality for most European capitals with their respective national rates (Bardsley, 1999). Once again, this comparison provides supporting evidence for the "sick city" hypothesis. For example, on average, mortality rates for infants (0–4 years) are 7 percent higher in European capital cities than in their nations as a whole. In five cities, however, mortality rates are lower than the national average; these cities are Helsinki (–18%), Lisbon (–9%), Lazio (–12%), Madrid (–20%), and Lyon (–25%). This casts some doubt on the hypothesis that urban health is necessarily worse than national averages.

What about world cities such as New York, Paris, and London? Available data on infant mortality and life expectancy indicate that there is no urban health penalty and perhaps even a qualified advantage for these city residents. This advantage appears to be decisive across all three cities with respect to life expectancy at the age of 65. Such findings, however intriguing, do not refute the hypothesis that cities are unhealthy, for the strongest case has yet to be made—the case that these wealthy world cities, along with all other megacities, are places where flagrant inequalities exist among neighborhoods and subpopulation groups. All of the averages we have considered mask pockets of poverty with disadvantaged groups that have disproportionately poor health status.

THE HEALTHY CITY

The case for the healthy city is typically grounded in economic arguments or celebrations of the city's vitality and innovation in such diverse realms as architecture, urban design, culture, technology, and more. For example, President Clinton's State of the Union message in 1998 refers to U.S. cities as the "vibrant hubs of great metropolitan regions" (Clinton, 1998). Indeed, between 1982 and 1998, metropolitan areas in the United States generated 85 percent of all jobs and 86 percent of the nation's total economic growth. This economic power is concentrated among some regional giants that dwarf not only their own states but also most of the world's nations. Metropolitan New York's economic output, for example, is greater than that of 45 of the 50 states (HUD, 1998).

Claims for the enduring power of cities, including big cities, often come from the literature on urban planning and do not typically invoke measures of population health. But there is also some evidence from public health studies in support of the hypothesis that urban health compares favorably with that of the nation as a whole. The National Health Interview Survey, for example, is one of the most reliable indicators of perceived functional health in the United States. In contrast to the *Big City Health Inventory* (National Association of City and County Health Officials, 2007), which relies on outcome measures of health, the National Health Interview Survey suggests that most indicators of self-assessed health status are better in major metropolitan areas than for the country as a whole.

Beyond these comparisons of metropolitan areas, there is also evidence from the literature on urban and rural differences that supports the urban advantage hypothesis (Liff, Chow, and Greenberg, 1991; Mainous and Kohrs, 1995). We can conclude, then, that while there is clearly evidence of an "urban penalty" in the United States, there is also evidence of an "urban advantage" in terms of self-assessed health status, health habits, and high-quality cancer screening services. What is more, among the three world cities we examine in this book, there appears to be an urban advantage for persons 65 years or older.

MAKING SENSE OF THE EVIDENCE

A selective review of evidence can support the urban advantage hypothesis. There is insufficient evidence, however, to provide strong support for either the urban health penalty or the urban health advantage hypothesis. The reason we have so little solid evidence is that there are no information collection systems for routine monitoring of the health of populations living in cities. While institutions responsible for disease surveillance—at the international, the national, and the local authority levels—collect vital statistics and epidemiologic data by geographic location, most nations make national health policy decisions without systematic analysis of the information about health status, public health infrastructure, and the performance of health systems in cities.

The rationale for comparing New York, Paris, and London is to illustrate the extent of variation in health status, health systems, and public health infrastructure among cities that share important characteristics and problems in so many other respects (Rodwin and Gusmano, 2002). Although this analysis also illustrates many of the difficulties of finding comparable data across relevant spatial units and time periods, it is nevertheless a good starting point because these cities have some of the most extensive databases available anywhere.

Variations in Access to Health Services among Residents of World Cities

OVERALL HEALTH SYSTEM PERFORMANCE

Avoidable mortality measures deaths before the age of 75 due to diseases for which there are effective health care interventions. There were significant declines in the rates of avoidable mortality in all three nations and urban cores during the 1990s. Manhattan experienced the greatest decline in the rate of avoidable mortality (20%) in comparison to Paris (16%) and Inner London (13%). Since the early 1990s, Manhattan, Paris, and Inner London have all placed great emphasis on primary and secondary prevention efforts to address diseases that represent the leading causes of avoidable mortality, so it is possible that these efforts help to explain the reductions during the 1990s. Yet, as we argued in Chapter 3, while the changes we observe may be due to public health interventions, they may also be the result of changes in the populations of these cities. With this caveat in mind, we believe our comparison of avoidable mortality among and within these urban cores provides insights into the performance of these three systems.

Although Manhattan as a whole has lower rates of avoidable mortality than Inner London and was able to reduce overall rates of avoidable mortality more than Paris or Inner London during the 1990s, inequality of access to timely and effective health care appears to be a much greater problem in Manhattan than in Paris or Inner London, where there is universal access to health care coverage. Those living in the lowest-income areas of Manhattan exhibit significantly higher rates of avoidable mortality than people living in the rest of the borough.

ACCESS TO PRIMARY CARE

In the United States, lack of timely, effective primary care, attributable largely to inadequate health insurance coverage, often results in unnecessary illness, loss of productivity, and costly hospitalizations that could be prevented. It is difficult to quantify the magnitude of unnecessary illness and loss of productivity. But our comparison of Manhattan, Paris, and Inner London documents some important consequences of access barriers in a city that is known for its strong health care safety net institutions. In Manhattan, the rate of admissions for avoidable hospital conditions is considerably higher than in Paris or Inner London, where all residents benefit from systems with universal health care coverage that effectively eliminate financial barriers to health care. Although our findings suggest that insurance is only one of several barriers to care in Manhattan, it is clearly important.

ACCESS TO SPECIALTY CARE

Our findings regarding hospital discharge rates, by area of patient residence, for acute myocardial infarction (AMI) as well as ischemic heart disease (IHD) are consistent with previous cross-national comparisons of heart disease in France and the United States. Death rates are higher in the United States and Manhattan than in France and Paris. Likewise, hospital discharge rates for AMI and all IHD provide strong evidence that the burden of IHD is significantly higher in the United States and Manhattan than in France and Paris. The disparity in disease burden between the United States and France, and Manhattan and Paris, increases with age, and mortality rates from all IHD are more than three times higher in the United States and Manhattan than in France and Paris.

A recent comparison of trends in the use of invasive procedures for patients with heart disease indicates that the United States has higher rates of cardiac catheterization, percutaneous transluminal coronary angioplasty (PTCA), and coronary artery bypass graft (CABG) surgery within one year after a heart attack than the other high-income OECD nations in the study (Technological Change in Health Care Research Network, 2001). Similarly, a comparison of the United States and Canada in the GUSTO-1 study found that the rates of PTCA and CABG among Canadian patients following AMI were much lower than any of the regional rates reported for the United States (Rouleau et al., 1993).

When we adjust for the burden of disease in the United States, France, England, and their world cities, the contrast between our findings and those of previous comparisons are striking. At the national level, the rate of revascularization among persons 65 years or older is actually highest for residents of France. Although the rate is lowest among residents of England for all age groups, the differences we find are much smaller than previous studies suggest.

After adjusting for the burden of disease in our urban cores, Parisians have a higher rate of revascularization than residents of Manhattan for all age groups. The rate of revascularization is lowest among residents of Inner London, but the difference is smaller than those found by the studies cited earlier, which are based on national data alone. Our findings underscore the possibility that many people who need these procedures in Manhattan may fail to receive them. Such a finding illustrates the added value of supplementing cross-national studies with city-level comparisons and appears entirely consistent with the characterization of the U.S. health care system as one marked by "excess and deprivation" (Enthoven and Kronick, 1989).

THE DISTRIBUTION OF CARE WITHIN MANHATTAN, PARIS, AND INNER LONDON

In Manhattan, we find much larger gaps in access by neighborhood socio-economic status than in our other urban cores. Some of this is due to the more significant geographic concentration of poverty (and lower rates of health insurance coverage) in Manhattan. Race-based residential segregation and the geographic concentration of poverty among blacks in Manhattan contribute to disparities in population health and disparities in access to services (Schulz et al., 2002; Weisz and Gusmano, 2006). Our findings in this study suggest that universal health care coverage alone is insufficient to eliminate geographic inequities in access to care. Nevertheless, it is seems clear that universal coverage would reduce disparities in access to primary care by at least reducing the financial barrier to health care.

Health care resources are typically distributed unequally in cities, reflecting the unequal distribution of wealth, income, and other goods and services (Andrulis, 1997; Fossett and Perloff, 1995; Politzer et al., 1991). This is particularly true in Manhattan; there are high concentrations of health and social services in areas where high-income-yielding jobs are most dense and in those neighborhoods where most residents work in these jobs (Lantz et al., 1998). The combination of these patterns of employment distribution along with significant financial barriers to health care—unique to the U.S. health care system—help explain why the age-adjusted rate of avoidable mortality is related significantly to income levels in the neighborhood of residence in Manhattan, but not in the other cities.

Unlike in Paris or Inner London, residents of the lowest-income neighborhoods in Manhattan are less likely to obtain access to timely and effective health care. In these neighborhoods, a large percentage of the population is either underinsured or uninsured. As a result, they face substantial financial barriers to access. In addition, residents of these neighborhoods are less likely to have a regular source of medical care. As we have shown in Chapters 4 and 5, even after controlling for insurance and race or ethnicity, the neighborhood of residence is correlated significantly with access to primary and specialty care.

Health Policy and City Limits

Our analysis documents that poor and other vulnerable populations face barriers to health care in all of three cities, with the greatest barriers in Manhattan. New York City's health care safety net is one of the largest in the world, and its Department of Health and Mental Hygiene has been aggressive and innovative in its efforts to improve the health of city residents. As we argued earlier, however, the growth in the number of uninsured and the increasing immigration and ethnic diversity of the city make this challenge even more daunting.

We should not underestimate a city government's ability to address social issues, including the health of its residents (Peterson, 1981; Stone, 1989). Nor should we overestimate the capacity of welfare states to serve those who fall through the cracks of a host of health and social entitlement programs. But cities are limited in their ability to redistribute income and address neighborhood-level poverty, inequality, and access to health care (Judd and Swanstrom, 1994). Cities, and other local governments, are left to cope with the many social problems, including the health and well-being of older residents, that are not addressed adequately by the federal and state governments.

Nevertheless, urban theory suggests that cities are limited by competition for mobile capital (Stone, 1989: xi). As a result of this competition, politicians, citizens, and economic elites often pursue development policies that enhance the economic productivity of the city (Jones and Bachelor, 1986: 8). Some argue that the economic imperatives faced by cities make it impossible for city policy makers to redistribute income or address the needs of their most vulnerable residents (Peterson, 1981). Others, however, suggest that it is possible to build a coalition around human capital development.

In a study of Baltimore, Orr (1992) chronicles the long and difficult battle fought by a strong community-based organization, Baltimoreans United in Leadership Development (BUILD), to place education policy on the political agenda. It is often difficult to build a coalition around human capital development, but through negotiation and compromise, relationships are established that aid each sector of the community in carrying out its particular agenda. Likewise, by using a combination of training, research, and confrontation, BUILD was able to forge a coalition with the business community and subsequently gain the support of then mayoral candidate Kurt Schmoke around their education proposals. The most crucial elements in the establishment of this relationship were a mayor who was willing to use his formal and informal powers to promote the issue and the ability of an organization based on expanding the opportunities of Baltimore's lower-class citizens to pressure the business community into supporting its plan (Orr, 1992).

The possibility of developing a coalition in support of human capital development and the ability of city mayors to influence levels of crime, education, health care, and other goals does not mean that mayors can work miracles (Judd and Swanstrom, 1994: 388). The geographic, financial, racial, and ethnic barriers to health care documented in this book are not primarily the result of city policies, and cities do not have the fiscal or legal capacity to overcome them. The problems we document help us better understand the consequences of national health and social policies— not the least of which is the failure to invest in cities or pay serious attention to the challenges they face (Crane, 2008).

Summary

The findings from our analysis of health care in world cities inform the current debate over health care reform in the United States, in which considerations of health systems abroad with universal coverage are routinely mischaracterized. Advocates for a "single-payer" system (a peculiar term that is rarely defined and serves primarily as a metaphor for universal coverage) dismiss the problems faced by other health care systems and lionize their positive attributes. Critics of "government-run" systems with universal coverage often imply that all such systems are like the English National Health Service, with severe limits on health care spending that result in waiting lists (although these have fallen dramatically in recent years; see Leatherman and Sutherland, 2008), and other "unacceptable" forms of "rationing." More sophisticated accounts suggest that health systems with universal coverage provide better access to primary care and are more equitable than the system in United States, but fail to provide the same level of access to specialty services (Goodman, Musgrave, and Herrick, 2004). Such caricatures of health systems abroad can be supported— but only through selective use of the evidence.

Our analysis documents significant variation among world cities in three nations: the United States, France, and the United Kingdom. In contrast to the United States, France and the United Kingdom have, respectively, a national health insurance system and a national health service, both of which provide universal coverage to their resident populations— yet do so with different levels of funding, distinct institutional structures, and contrasting opportunities for access to different levels of health care. If learning from different health systems requires, at a minimum, accurately portraying the systems at stake (Marmor, Freeman, and Okma, 2005), we need to move beyond simplistic characterizations and develop more sophisticated methods for assessing and extending the specific dimensions of health care access, some of which we have sought to demonstrate in this book.

The three world cities we have examined in this book enjoy extraordinary health care resources but face significant health care inequalities. Although New York City's health care safety net is one of the largest in the world and its Department of Health and Mental Hygiene has been aggressive and innovative in its efforts to improve the health of city residents, the health care inequalities we document in the preceding chapters are greatest in Manhattan. National policies have left large numbers of Americans without health insurance and have produced a geographic concentration of poverty in our cities' poorest neighborhoods. These policies place a burden on New York City that Paris and London do not share.

In reflecting on utopia, George Bernard Shaw once quipped, "Some men see things as they are and ask why. Others dream of things that never were and ask why not." In this book, we have focused on health systems in three world cities "as they are." Along with analyzing their relative performance with respect to reducing avoidable deaths and providing access to primary, as well as specialty care, we hope that our comparisons will provoke some deliberation as to how "things" might improve. As we noted at the outset (Chapter 1), an initial goal of our project was to reflect on the consequences of poor access to health care in New York, London, and Paris and the broader health systems of which they are a part. Unlike Shaw, we do not suggest that policy makers must "dream of things that never were," but we hope they will not limit their vision to seeing things only "as they are." The problems of inequitable access to health care in Manhattan could no doubt be documented in many more cities throughout the United States. The comparison among the urban cores of our three world cities suggests that similar places share our problems—yet the extent of inequalities evident in Manhattan is not inevitable. Recognizing that the way things are is not the way they have to be is surely insufficient to effect change, but a necessary and useful first step.

APPENDIX
Data and Methods

Data Sources

Population Data

We used population data by cohorts from the Bureau of the Census for the United States, from the Institut National de la Statistique et des Etudes Economiques (INSEE) for France, and from the Office of National Statistics for England.

Hospital Administrative Data

Our hospital discharge data for calculating avoidable hospital conditions and revascularizations came from the following sources:

- *United States*: Hospital discharge data from the National Hospital Discharge Survey, National Center for Health Statistics (NCHS).
- *New York City*: Hospital discharge data from the Statewide Planning and Resource Cooperative System (SPARCS), which includes information for all residents of Manhattan discharged from all nonfederal hospitals in New York State, excluding the population cared for in Veterans Administration hospitals.
- *France and Paris*: The French Ministry of Health's Programme de Médicalisation des Systèmes d'Information (PMSI). PMSI centralizes hospital discharge data by diagnosis, procedure, age, and residence of patients. It includes data from all hospitals (public and private) of more than 100 beds, thus possibly excluding a very small number of discharges for avoidable hospital conditions (AHCs) in Paris.
- *England and London*: Hospital Episode Statistics (HES) data on patients treated in the National Health Service (NHS) from the Department of Health and Social Security (DHSS). HES includes information for all residents of Inner London on all hospitalizations, in NHS hospitals as well as private hospitals, paid for by the NHS.

The city-level hospital discharge data are for residents of all three cities irrespective of whether they were hospitalized within or outside these cities.

To conduct our analysis we relied on the following data elements from these datasets.

- *From SPARCS:* (1) Zip code, (2) age, (3) sex, (4) race, (5) ethnicity, (6) date of birth, (7) principal diagnosis (International Classification of Diseases-9), (8) all other diagnoses (ICD-9), (9) admission date, (10) discharge date, (11) same-day discharge indicator, (12) length of stay, (13) primary reimbursement code, (14) secondary reimbursement code.
- *From PMSI:* (1) Arrondissement (Paris zip code), (2) age, (3) sex, (4) principal diagnosis (ICD-10), (5) secondary diagnoses (ICD-10), (6) discharge destination, (7) same-day discharge indicator.
- *From HES:* (1) Borough, (2) ward, (3) seven-digit postal code, (4) primary care trust code, (5) age, (6) sex, (7) ethnicity, (8) principal diagnosis (ICD-10), (9) secondary diagnoses (ICD-10), (10) discharge destination, (11) same-day discharge indicator.

International Classification of Disease Codes

The International Classification of Diseases (ICD) was developed collaboratively between the World Health Organization (WHO) and ten international centers, including the NCHS. The ICD has been revised infrequently, and there was a 20-year interval between the last two revisions, ICD-9 and ICD-10. ICD-10 is currently being introduced in the United States.

ICD-10 is more detailed than ICD-9 (for example, it has 8,000 valid categories for cause of death compared with 4,000 in ICD-9). Much of the expansion was intended to provide more detail for morbidity applications. ICD-10 employs four-digit alphanumeric codes instead of the four-digit numeric codes in ICD-9. There are also three additional chapters in ICD-10, and some chapters have been rearranged. The available conversion tables compare equivalent categories but are only approximate because, for most categories, ICD-10 is more detailed than ICD-9. To ensure continuity in choosing the relevant diagnostic codes, we sought guidance from physicians and trained medical coders in all three cities.

Mortality Data

To calculate avoidable and total mortality, we used publicly available mortality data by the following age cohorts: 1–4, 5–14, 15–24, 25–34, 35–44, 45–54, 55–64, and 65–74. We obtained data on causes of death coded according to ICD-9 or ICD-10, for selected geographic areas.

For New York City and the United States, we extracted data from National Vital Statistics Reports published by the NCHS Division of the Centers for Disease Control and Prevention (CDC). For Paris and France, we used mortality data from the Institut National de la Santé et de Recherche Médicale (INSERM). For London and England, we used data from the National Office of Statistics.

National Health Statistics

The sources for national health statistics, by city and country, were the following:

- New York City and the United States: NCHS/CDC
- London and England: Office of National Statistics, London Health Observatory
- Paris and France: Institut national de la statistique et des études économiques (INSEE), Observatoire Regional de la Santé de l'Ile de France

Health System Data

Our sources for health system data were as follows:

- New York City and the United States: United Hospital Fund's *Health Care Annual*; New York State Department of Health
- Paris and France: Direction Régionale des Affaires Sanitaires et Sociales d'Île de France; Ministère de l'Emploi et de la Solidarité, Service des Statistiques des Études et des Systèmes d'Information (SESI), repertoire ADELI au 1er janvier 98
- London and England: London Health Observatory; Department of Health

Data Analysis

Regression Analysis of Avoidable Hospitalization
Conditions and Revascularization

We used logistic regression analysis to identify the factors associated with the dependent variables for avoidable hospital conditions (AHCs) and revascularization. For AHCs, we used the following model:

$$Ln\left(\frac{Pr(AHC_{il})}{Pr(AHC_{ii})}\right) = \alpha + \sum_{k-1}^{k} B_1 Age + B_2 Gender + B_3 NumDiag_t + \eta SES$$
$$+ \iota Education + \kappa Physicians + \lambda HospitalBeds$$

The independent individual variables in this model and the next one are age, gender, race/ethnicity, primary payers, and number of diagnoses on the record (as a measure of severity of illness); the neighborhood variables are indicators for income quartile and physician density. For Manhattan and Inner London, we used an individual-level variable for race/ethnicity, but in France, it is illegal to collect information about race/ethnicity, so we were unable to include this variable in our Paris models.

To analyze the use of revascularization, we limited the analysis to those hospitalized with some form of ischemic heart disease (IHD) and relied on the following model:

$$Ln\left(\frac{\Pr(Revasc_{it})}{\Pr(\overline{Revasc}_{it})}\right) = \alpha + \sum_{k-1}^{k} B_1 AgeSquared + B_2 Gender + B_3 NumDiag + \eta SES$$
$$+ \kappa Education + \lambda Physicians + \mu HospitalBeds$$

To predict revascularization, we also included the variable "age squared" in our models, in addition to continuous age variables, because the probability of revascularization increases between the ages of 35 and 75, but decreases thereafter due to increasing frailty. To illustrate the relationship between age and revascularization, Figure A.1 is based on data from Manhattan.

Because observations on individuals from the same geographic area may be correlated, we tested for bias due to unobserved neighborhood-level heterogeneity by estimating the models with a dummy variable for each zip code as a replacement for neighborhood-level variables (Greene, 2000). We also ran full models with secondary payers, as well as interactive terms relating race and area income, and race and insurance. In addition to examining models with dummy variables, we used STATA (version 8) to examine the variance inflation factor (VIF) as a test of collinearity (STATA command: collin). Because the VIF is less than 10 for all of our independent variables, we concluded that the correlations among them are

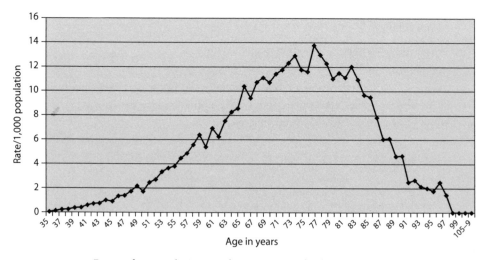

FIG. A.1. Rates of revascularization, by age, in Manhattan, 1998–2002.

not causing unacceptable biases. (For further discussion of VIF, see Greene, 2000.) The findings from these alternative models were not appreciably different from the models we present in the chapters.

Regression Analysis of Amenable Mortality

To investigate the extent to which there are geographic disparities in avoidable mortality among our urban core neighborhoods, we estimated the relationship between area income and the percentage of avoidable deaths using OLS regression. Because avoidable deaths are a rare occurrence, are a non-negative count variable, and exhibit greater variation than in a true Poisson process, we used a negative binomial regression model to test the null hypothesis that there are no differences in rates of avoidable mortality between low-income and higher-income neighborhoods. The number of deaths is the response, the population less than 75 years of age is the exposure, and the income-related indicator is the explanatory variable. We have not reported the estimate of the underlying coefficient of the income variable but only the exponential of the estimate, the estimated incident rate ratio (IRR). This is the ratio of the value of the avoidable mortality rate in the low-income areas to that in the other states, counties, or zip codes. Our null hypothesis was that the IRR is 1, that there is no difference in mortality between the higher- and lower-income areas. The alternative hypothesis was that the IRR exceeds 1, which indicates that lower-income areas have higher avoidable mortality rates than the higher-income areas.

Analytic Issues and Limitations

We calculated rates of AHCs, revascularization, and mortality from acute myocardial infarction (AMI) for age-adjusted cohorts, employing the direct standardization method and using the U.N.'s 2005 world population estimate to obtain adjustment weights.

Our index of the rate of revascularization to the rate of AMI mortality does not assume that every person who has an AMI should receive one of these procedures. Nor do we assume that this is the only diagnosis for which these procedures are appropriate. Our index is merely an attempt to adjust for the different burden of disease among these nations. It is possible that mortality rates do not adequately capture morbidity. We therefore conducted a sensitivity analysis in which we substituted other measures of disease burden in the denominator of our index (mortality due to all coronary heart disease, all ischemic heart disease, and hospitalizations for these conditions). The results did not change greatly when we used these alternative measures of heart disease. The one exception was the use of hospitalization for AMI in the denominator for England. Although mortality rates for AMI are about 20 percent higher in England than in the United States, hospital discharge rates for AMI are more than 40 percent lower. This suggests that many people whose deaths are attributed to AMI are not admitted to hospital in England. We therefore consider mortality rates a more reliable proxy for the burden of disease, particularly in England. While our index is limited by available data, failure to consider some measure of disease burden when analyzing treatment rates is clearly misleading.

Because we did not examine clinical data, we were unable to comment on the appropriateness of care. Although there is evidence that some patients who receive revascularization in United States do not benefit from it (Senior, 2006), other studies find that many people who need these procedures fail to receive them because of lack of insurance and other nonclinical barriers to medical care, including race (Popescu, Vaughan-Sarrazin, and Rosenthal, 2007). Hence, it is possible that the average rates for the United States as well as for our other countries include both over- and underuse.

Summary Statistics

TABLE A.I. Rates of avoidable hospital conditions in Manhattan and its United Hospital Fund (UHF) neighborhoods, 1999–2001

Area (UHF neighborhood)	N	Age-specific rate per 1,000 population	Age-adjusted rate per 1,000 population
All Manhattan	17,400	14.2	16.1
Washington Heights	2,861	14.8	16.8
Central Harlem	2,453	22.8	24.6
East Harlem	2,579	34.5	36.6
Upper West Side	2,010	10.8	11.5
Upper East Side	1,606	8.5	9.0
Chelsea/Clinton	1,417	12.7	15.4
Gramercy Park / Murray Hill	1,606	8.5	9.0
Greenwich Village / SoHo	1,417	12.7	15.4
Union Square / Lower East Side	1,069	9.4	10.6
Lower Manhattan	566	7.6	9.9
Mean		14.2	15.9
Standard error		2.7	2.8
Median		11.8	13.4
Standard deviation		8.4	8.7
Sample variance		70.6	76.0
Kurtosis		3.5	3.1
Skewness		1.9	1.8
Range		26.9	27.6
Minimum		7.6	9.0
Maximum		34.5	36.6
Ratio max/min		4.5	4.1
Count		10.0	10.0
Confidence level (95.0%)		6.0	6.2

TABLE A.2. Rates of marker conditions with acute myocardial infarction for persons age 20 and above in Manhattan and its UHF neighborhoods, 1999–2001

Area (UHF neighborhood)	N	Age-specific rate per 1,000 population	Age-adjusted rate per 1,000 population
All Manhattan	4,988	4.1	4.7
Washington Heights	727	3.8	4.3
Central Harlem	395	3.7	4.0
East Harlem	396	5.3	5.7
Upper West Side	750	4.0	4.3
Upper East Side	799	4.2	4.5
Chelsea/Clinton	477	4.3	5.2
Gramercy Park / Murray Hill	442	3.9	4.4
Greenwich Village / SoHo	206	2.8	3.5
Union Square / Lower East Side	685	4.3	4.6
Lower Manhattan	99	4.0	4.7
Mean		4.0	4.5
Standard error		0.2	0.2
Median		4.0	4.4
Standard deviation		0.6	0.6
Sample variance		0.4	0.4
Kurtosis		2.8	0.8
Skewness		0.1	0.5
Range		2.5	2.2
Minimum		2.8	3.5
Maximum		5.3	5.7
Ratio max/min		1.9	1.6
Count		10.0	10.0
Confidence level (95.0%)		0.5	0.4

TABLE A.3. Rates of acute myocardial infarction as primary hospital diagnosis for persons age 35 and above in Manhattan and its UHF neighborhoods, 1999–2001

Area (UHF neighborhood)	N	Age-specific rate per 1,000 population	Age-adjusted rate per 1,000 population
All Manhattan	1,953	2.5	2.7
Washington Heights	340	2.7	2.9
Central Harlem	180	2.6	2.6
East Harlem	190	3.9	3.9
Upper West Side	272	2.2	2.2
Upper East Side	243	2.0	1.9
Chelsea/Clinton	191	2.7	3.1
Gramercy Park / Murray Hill	149	2.1	2.1
Greenwich Village / SoHo	69	1.5	1.7
Union Square / Lower East Side	281	2.8	2.8
Lower Manhattan	33	2.3	2.4
Mean		2.5	2.6
Standard error		0.2	0.2
Median		2.4	2.5
Standard deviation		0.6	0.6
Sample variance		0.4	0.4
Kurtosis		2.2	1.0
Skewness		1.0	0.9
Range		2.4	2.2
Minimum		1.5	1.7
Maximum		3.9	3.9
Ratio max/min		2.5	2.3
Count		10.0	10.0
Confidence level (95.0%)		0.5	0.5

TABLE A.4. Rates of revascularization (PTCA+CABG coded in procedures 1–5) for persons age 35 and above diagnosed with ischemic heart disease in Manhattan and its UHF neighborhoods, 1999–2001

Area (UHF neighborhood)	N	Age-specific rate per 1,000 population	Age-adjusted rate per 1,000 population	Ratio of revascularization rate to AMI rate
All Manhattan	3,282	4.2	4.4	1.7
Washington Heights	380	3.1	3.3	1.1
Central Harlem	222	3.2	3.2	1.2
East Harlem	274	5.6	5.5	1.4
Upper West Side	514	4.2	4.3	2.0
Upper East Side	627	5.2	5.0	2.6
Chelsea/Clinton	290	4.2	4.7	1.5
Gramercy Park / Murray Hill	334	4.8	4.6	2.2
Greenwich Village / SoHo	147	3.2	3.6	2.1
Union Square / Lower East Side	435	4.3	4.3	1.6
Lower Manhattan	49	3.4	3.6	1.5
Mean		4.1	4.2	1.7
Standard error		0.3	0.2	0.1
Median		4.2	4.3	1.5
Standard deviation		0.9	0.8	0.5
Sample variance		0.8	0.6	0.2
Kurtosis		−1.1	−1.0	−0.5
Skewness		0.4	0.2	0.6
Range		2.5	2.3	1.5
Minimum		3.1	3.2	1.1
Maximum		5.6	5.5	2.6
Ratio max/min		1.8	1.7	2.3
Count		10.0	10.0	10.0
		0.6	0.6	0.3

TABLE A.5. Rates of all hospital admissions for persons age 18 and above in Manhattan and its UHF neighborhoods, 1999–2001

Area (UHF neighborhood)	N	Age-specific rate per 1,000 population	Age-adjusted rate per 1,000 population
All Manhattan	160,284	130.5	142.4
Washington Heights	25,203	130.4	139.3
Central Harlem	19,631	182.8	191.5
East Harlem	17,721	237.2	248.0
Upper West Side	20,371	109.0	114.5
Upper East Side	19,481	103.3	106.7
Chelsea/Clinton	14,494	130.3	148.2
Gramercy Park / Murray Hill	13,184	115.4	126.6
Greenwich Village / SoHo	5,937	80.0	95.0
Union Square / Lower East Side	20,714	128.5	137.2
Lower Manhattan	2,918	117.1	131.3
Mean		133.4	143.8
Standard error		14.2	14.3
Median		122.8	134.2
Standard deviation		45.0	45.1
Sample variance		2,022.4	2,032.2
Kurtosis		2.7	2.6
Skewness		1.6	1.6
Range		157.2	153.0
Minimum		80.0	95.0
Maximum		237.2	248.0
Ratio max/min		3.0	2.6
Count		10.0	10.0
Confidence level (95.0%)		32.2	32.2

TABLE A.6. Rates of avoidable hospital conditions in Paris and its arrondissements, 1999–2001

Area (arrondissement)	N	Age-specific rate per 1,000 population	Age-adjusted rate per 1,000 population
All Paris	17,211	9.9	9.5
75001	168	11.6	11.8
75002	148	8.8	10.3
75003	244	8.5	9.6
75004	249	9.4	9.0
75005	376	7.6	7.0
75006	284	7.6	6.3
75007	399	8.4	6.8
75008	261	8.2	7.3
75009	422	9.1	9.1
75010	784	10.8	11.9
75011	1,184	9.5	10.3
75012	1,113	9.9	9.1
75013	1,389	10.0	9.9
75014	1,067	9.6	9.0
75015	1,629	8.6	7.8
75016	1,218	9.3	7.1
75017	1,199	9.1	8.3
75018	1,732	11.5	11.9
75019	1,626	12.4	12.9
75020	1,656	11.4	11.5
Mean		9.5	9.3
Standard error		0.3	0.4
Median		9.3	9.1
Standard deviation		1.4	2.0
Sample variance		1.9	3.8
Kurtosis		−0.4	−0.9
Skewness		0.6	0.2
Range		4.8	6.7
Minimum		7.6	6.3
Maximum		12.4	12.9
Ratio max/min		1.6	2.1
Count		20.0	20.0
Confidence level (95.0%)		0.6	0.9

TABLE A.7. Rates of marker conditions with acute myocardial infarction for persons age 20 and above in Paris and its arrondissements, 1999–2001

Area (arrondissement)	N	Age-specific rate per 1,000 population	Age-adjusted rate per 1,000 population
All Paris	8,096	4.7	4.3
75001	126	8.7	8.1
75002	67	4.0	4.3
75003	113	3.9	4.3
75004	108	4.1	3.8
75005	208	4.2	3.6
75006	175	4.6	3.8
75007	233	4.9	3.7
75008	148	4.7	4.1
75009	209	4.5	4.3
75010	316	4.4	4.6
75011	543	4.4	4.5
75012	566	5.0	4.3
75013	587	4.2	4.1
75014	527	4.7	4.2
75015	867	4.6	4.0
75016	706	5.4	3.9
75017	619	4.7	4.0
75018	683	4.6	4.5
75019	578	4.4	4.6
75020	677	4.7	4.6
Mean		4.7	4.4
Standard error		0.2	0.2
Median		4.6	4.2
Standard deviation		1.0	0.9
Sample variance		1.0	0.9
Kurtosis		14.7	15.3
Skewness		3.6	3.7
Range		4.8	4.5
Minimum		3.9	3.6
Maximum		8.7	8.1
Ratio max/min		2.2	2.3
Count		20.0	20.0
Confidence level (95.0%)		0.5	0.4

TABLE A.8. Rates of acute myocardial infarction as primary hospital diagnosis for persons age 35 and above in Paris and its arrondissements, 1999–2001

Area (arrondissement)	N	Age-specific rate per 1,000 population	Age-adjusted rate per 1,000 population
All Paris	1,786	1.6	1.4
75001	18	2.0	1.7
75002	13	1.3	1.4
75003	30	1.8	1.7
75004	28	1.7	1.4
75005	44	1.5	1.2
75006	38	1.5	1.2
75007	47	1.4	1.1
75008	34	1.6	1.4
75009	46	1.5	1.4
75010	75	1.7	1.6
75011	140	1.8	1.8
75012	126	1.7	1.4
75013	150	1.6	1.5
75014	104	1.5	1.3
75015	167	1.4	1.2
75016	132	1.4	1.1
75017	143	1.6	1.5
75018	136	1.4	1.3
75019	136	1.5	1.5
75020	177	1.8	1.7
Mean		1.6	1.4
Standard error		0.0	0.0
Median		1.6	1.4
Standard deviation		0.2	0.2
Sample variance		0.0	0.0
Kurtosis		0.3	−0.9
Skewness		0.7	0.2
Range		0.7	0.7
Minimum		1.3	1.1
Maximum		2.0	1.8
Ratio max/min		1.5	1.7
Count		20.0	20.0
Confidence level (95.0%)		0.1	0.1

TABLE A.9   Rates of revascularization (PTCA + CABG coded in procedures 1–5) for persons age 35 and above diagnosed with ischemic heart disease in Paris and its arrondissements, 1999–2001

Area (arrondissement)	N	Age-specific rate per 1,000 population	Age-adjusted rate per 1,000 population	Ratio of revascular- ization rate to AMI rate
All Paris	2,927	2.6	2.4	1.7
75001	30	3.3	3.1	1.8
75002	29	2.9	2.9	2.2
75003	37	2.2	2.2	1.3
75004	41	2.4	2.1	1.5
75005	77	2.5	2.2	1.9
75006	70	2.8	2.4	1.9
75007	104	3.2	2.6	2.3
75008	66	3.0	2.7	2.0
75009	66	2.2	2.2	1.6
75010	94	2.1	2.2	1.3
75011	185	2.4	2.4	1.3
75012	182	2.4	2.2	1.6
75013	256	2.8	2.6	1.7
75014	165	2.3	2.1	1.7
75015	300	2.5	2.2	1.9
75016	332	3.5	2.8	2.6
75017	219	2.5	2.3	1.6
75018	232	2.4	2.4	1.8
75019	193	2.2	2.2	1.4
75020	239	2.4	2.4	1.4
Mean		2.6	2.4	1.7
Standard error		0.1	0.1	0.1
Median		2.5	2.3	1.7
Standard deviation		0.4	0.3	0.3
Sample variance		0.2	0.1	0.1
Kurtosis		−0.2	0.6	0.8
Skewness		0.8	1.2	0.9
Range		1.4	1.0	1.4
Minimum		2.1	2.1	1.3
Maximum		3.5	3.1	2.6
Ratio max/min		1.6	1.5	2.1
Count		20.0	20.0	20.0
Confidence level (95.0%)		0.2	0.1	0.2

TABLE A.10. Rates of all hospital admissions for persons age 20 and above in Paris and its arrondissements, 1999–2001

Area (arrondissement)	N	Age-specific rate per 1,000 population	Age-adjusted rate per 1,000 population
All Paris	296,370	170.6	167.8
75001	3,608	248.8	255.4
75002	2,716	162.4	176.7
75003	4,384	152.2	163.5
75004	4,146	156.9	154.8
75005	6,800	137.0	136.9
75006	5,445	144.8	135.8
75007	7,323	154.5	140.0
75008	4,989	157.4	151.2
75009	7,492	162.1	162.0
75010	12,670	174.3	184.7
75011	20,603	165.9	172.9
75012	19,953	176.8	170.6
75013	23,694	170.5	170.1
75014	18,681	167.3	166.0
75015	29,461	156.3	149.7
75016	21,615	164.3	145.7
75017	21,286	161.4	154.8
75018	27,271	181.8	184.4
75019	26,274	200.0	203.4
75020	26,650	184.2	184.9
Mean		168.9	168.2
Standard error		5.3	6.1
Median		163.3	164.8
Standard deviation		23.6	27.3
Sample variance		554.9	745.1
Kurtosis		6.6	4.7
Skewness		2.2	1.7
Range		111.8	119.7
Minimum		137.0	135.8
Maximum		248.8	255.4
Ratio max/min		1.8	1.9
Count		20.0	20.0
Confidence level (95.0%)		11.0	12.8

TABLE A.11. Rates of avoidable hospital conditions for persons age 20 and above in Inner London and its boroughs, 1999–2001

Area (borough)	N	Age-specific rate per 1,000 population	Age-adjusted rate per 1,000 population
Inner London	2,2021	10.5	12.7
City of London	53	12.2	9.0
Camden	1,612	11.1	12.4
Hackney	1,510	10.4	12.6
Hammersmith	1,476	11.2	13.8
Haringuey	1,435	8.9	10.8
Islington	1,548	11.4	14.4
Kensington	1,122	8.7	9.5
Lambeth	1,835	9.0	11.7
Lewisham	1,878	10.2	11.6
Newham	2,049	12.4	15.3
Southwark	1,838	10.0	12.1
Tower Hamlets	1,796	12.8	16.5
Wandsworth	1,843	8.8	11.0
Westminster	2,028	13.5	15.5
Mean		10.8	12.6
Standard error		0.4	0.6
Median		10.8	12.2
Standard deviation		1.6	2.3
Sample variance		2.5	5.1
Kurtosis		−1.1	−0.8
Skewness		0.2	0.2
Range		4.8	7.6
Minimum		8.7	9.0
Maximum		13.5	16.5
Ratio max/min		1.6	1.8
Count		14.0	14.0
Confidence level (95.0%)		0.9	1.3

TABLE A.12. Rates of marker conditions with acute myocardial infarction for persons age 20 and above in Inner London and its boroughs, 1999–2001

Area (borough)	N	Age-specific rate per 1,000 population	Age-adjusted rate per 1,000 population
Inner London	8,182	3.9	4.8
City of London	22	5.0	3.7
Camden	632	4.4	5.0
Hackney	546	3.8	4.7
Hammersmith	499	3.8	4.7
Haringuey	574	3.6	4.5
Islington	573	4.2	5.5
Kensington	430	3.3	3.7
Lambeth	600	2.9	4.0
Lewisham	737	4.0	4.5
Newham	739	4.5	5.8
Southwark	607	3.3	4.1
Tower Hamlets	621	4.4	6.2
Wandsworth	786	3.8	4.7
Westminster	818	5.5	6.3
Mean		4.0	4.8
Standard error		0.2	0.2
Median		3.9	4.7
Standard deviation		0.7	0.8
Sample variance		0.5	0.7
Kurtosis		0.1	−0.7
Skewness		0.5	0.5
Range		2.5	2.6
Minimum		2.9	3.7
Maximum		5.5	6.3
Ratio max/min		1.9	1.7
Count		14.0	14.0
Confidence level (95.0%)		0.4	0.5

TABLE A.13. Rates of acute myocardial infarction as primary hospital diagnosis for persons age 35 and above in Inner London and its boroughs, 1999–2001

Area (borough)	N	Age-specific rate per 1,000 population	Age-adjusted rate per 1,000 population
Inner London	3,068	1.5	2.7
City of London	7	1.6	1.7
Camden	205	1.4	2.4
Hackney	221	2.5	2.8
Hammersmith	185	2.5	2.6
Haringuey	224	2.3	2.5
Islington	217	2.7	2.9
Kensington	139	1.7	1.7
Lambeth	201	1.8	2.0
Lewisham	298	2.6	2.7
Newham	398	4.0	4.4
Southwark	186	1.7	1.8
Tower Hamlets	236	3.2	3.2
Wandsworth	280	2.5	2.6
Westminster	273	3.1	3.0
Mean		2.4	2.6
Standard error		0.2	0.2
Median		2.5	2.6
Standard deviation		0.7	0.7
Sample variance		0.5	0.5
Kurtosis		0.2	1.8
Skewness		0.6	0.9
Range		2.6	2.7
Minimum		1.4	1.7
Maximum		4.0	4.4
Ratio max/min		2.9	2.6
Count		14.0	14.0
Confidence level (95.0%)		0.4	0.4

TABLE A.14. Rates of revascularization (PTCA + CABG coded in procedures 1–5) for persons age 35 and above diagnosed with ischemic heart disease in Inner London and its boroughs, 1999–2001

Area (Borough)	N	Age-specific rate per 1,000 population	Age-adjusted rate per 1,000 population	Ratio of revascularization rate to AMI rate
Inner London	2,424	1.2	2.1	0.8
City of London	7	1.6	1.6	1.0
Camden	175	1.2	2.0	0.8
Hackney	105	1.2	1.3	0.5
Hammersmith	160	2.2	2.3	0.9
Haringuey	122	1.3	1.3	0.5
Islington	110	1.4	1.4	0.5
Kensington	150	1.8	1.8	1.1
Lambeth	224	2.0	2.2	1.1
Lewisham	225	1.9	2.1	0.8
Newham	172	1.7	1.8	0.4
Southwark	240	2.2	2.3	1.3
Tower Hamlets	173	2.4	2.3	0.7
Wandsworth	226	2.0	2.1	0.8
Westminster	339	3.9	3.8	1.2
Mean		1.9	2.0	0.8
Standard error		0.2	0.2	0.1
Median		1.9	2.0	0.8
Standard deviation		0.7	0.6	0.3
Sample variance		0.5	0.4	0.1
Kurtosis		4.8	4.4	−1.1
Skewness		1.8	1.6	0.1
Range		2.7	2.5	0.9
Minimum		1.2	1.3	0.4
Maximum		3.9	3.8	1.3
Ratio max/min		3.2	2.9	3.1
Count		14.0	14.0	14.0
Confidence level (95.0%)		0.4	0.4	0.2

TABLE A.15. Rates of all hospital admissions for persons age 20 and above in Inner London and its boroughs, 1999–2001

Area (borough)	N	Age-specific rate per 1,000 population	Age-adjusted rate per 1,000 population
Inner London	518,687	246.7	277.0
City of London	1,137	263.0	192.8
Camden	37,467	258.3	268.9
Hackney	37,254	256.6	287.5
Hammersmith	30,402	230.0	266.2
Haringuey	40,992	253.9	280.0
Islington	35,362	260.0	301.2
Kensington	26,116	202.7	214.4
Lambeth	45,194	221.4	263.9
Lewisham	45,394	245.4	258.6
Newham	47,090	286.0	320.9
Southwark	44,538	242.0	269.7
Tower Hamlets	34,987	249.1	312.7
Wandsworth	44,722	214.0	247.7
Westminster	48,034	320.5	350.3
Mean		250.2	273.9
Standard error		7.9	10.9
Median		251.5	269.3
Standard deviation		29.7	40.9
Sample variance		884.4	1673.2
Kurtosis		1.4	0.4
Skewness		0.7	−0.2
Range		117.8	157.5
Minimum		202.7	192.8
Maximum		320.5	350.3
Ratio max/min		1.6	1.8
Count		14.0	14.0
Confidence level (95.0%)		17.2	23.6

Codes for Calculating Avoidable Mortality
and Avoidable Hospital Conditions

TABLE A.16. Conditions and ICD codes used to calculate avoidable mortality

Cause of death	ICD-9 codes	ICD-10 codes
Tuberculosis	010–018, 137	A15–19, B90
Septicemia	38	A40–41
Malignancy of colon and rectum	153–154	C18–21
Malignancy of skin	172–173	C44
Malignancy of breast	174–175	C50
Malignancy of cervix and uterus	179, 180, 182	C53–55
Malignancy of testis	186	C62
Hodgkin disease	201	C81
Leukemia	204–208	C91–95
Endocrine diseases, including diabetes mellitus	240–279	E0–69
Epilepsy	345	G40–41
Hypertension	401–405	I10–13
Cerebrovascular disease	430–438	I60–69
Influenza	487	J10–11
Pneumonia	480–486	J12–18
Ischemic heart disease	410–414	I20–25
Peptic ulcer	531–533	K25–27
Appendicitis, abdominal hernia, and gallbladder disease	540–543	K35–38
	550–553	K40–46
	574.0–575.1	K80–82
Nephritis and nephrosis	580–589	N0–7, 17–19, 25–27
Benign prostatic hyperplasia	600	N40
Maternal death	630–676	O00–99

TABLE A.17. Conditions and ICD codes used to calculate avoidable hospital conditions

Cause for admission	ICD-10 codes[a]
Immunizable conditions	A35–37, A80, B05, B25
Diabetes	E10.1, E10.64–10.65, E11.0, E11.64–11.65, E13.0–13.1, E13.64–13.65, E14.0–14.1, E14.64–14.65
Hypokalemia	E876
Congestive heart failure	I50
Hypertension	I10–15, I674
Pneumonia	J13–16, J18
Asthma	J45
Ruptured appendix	K35.0–35.1, K65.0, K65.8
Urinary infections (pyelonephritis)	N10–N12, 13.6, 15
Complications of peptic ulcer disease	K25.0–25.2, 25.4–25.6, K26.0–26.2, 26.4–26.6, K27.0–27.2, 27.4–27.6, K28.0–28.2, 28–28.6
Gangrene	R0.2, I73.9, I74.3
Cellulitis	L03.0–03.1, L03.8–03.9

SOURCE: Data from Weissman, Gatsonis, and Epstein, 1992

[a] The original definition of AHC by Weissman and colleagues (1992) relies on ICD-9. Of the 12 conditions included, 10 translate directly to ICD-10. Only two, pyelonephritis and gangrene, neither of which is a large contributor to the rate of AHCs, require interpretation. To capture pyelonephritis (ICD-9 codes 590.0, 590.1, and 590.8), we used ICD-10 codes N10–12, 13.6, and 15, which include pyelonephritis and acute and chronic tubulointerstitial nephritis and pyonephrosis. To capture all cases of gangrene included in ICD-9 785.4, we used R0.2 (gangrene unspecified), supplemented with I73.9 (unspecified peripheral vascular disease) and I74.3 (embolus and thrombosis of arteries of the lower extremity). These minor differences in coding have a negligible impact.

REFERENCES

Aaron, H. J., W. B. Schwartz, and M. Cox. 2005. *Can We Say No? The Challenge of Rationing Health Care.* Washington, DC: Brookings Institution Press.

AcademyHealth. 2007. *State of the States.* Washington, DC: AcademyHealth, January.

Aday, L. A., C. E. Begley, D. R. Lairson, and C. H. Slater. 1998. *Evaluating the Health Care System: Effectiveness, Efficacy, and Equity.* 2nd ed. Chicago: Health Administration Press.

AHA (American Heart Association). 2002. AHA guidelines for primary prevention of cardiovascular disease and stroke: 2002 update. *Circulation* 106:388.

Aicher, J. 1998. *Designing Healthy Cities: Prescriptions, Principles, and Practice.* Malabar, FL: Krieger Publishing.

Akosah, K. O., K. Moncher, A. Schaper, P. Havlik, and S. Devine. 2001. Chronic heart failure in the community: Missed diagnosis and missed opportunities. *Journal of Cardiac Failure* 7(3): 239–40.

Andersen, R. M. 1995. Revisiting the behavioral model and access to medical care: Does it matter? *Journal of Health and Social Behavior* 36 (March): 1–10.

Anderson, G., and J. Horvath. 2002. *Chronic Conditions: Making the Case for Ongoing Care.* Baltimore: Johns Hopkins University Press.

Anderson, G., and P. Hussey. 2001. Comparing health system performance in OECD countries. *Health Affairs* 20(3): 219–32.

Anderson, O. 1972. *Health Care: Can There Be Equity? The United States, Sweden, and England.* New York: John Wiley & Sons.

Andrulis, D. P. 1997. The urban health penalty: New dimensions and directions in inner-city health care. In *Inner-City Health Care.* Philadelphia: American College of Physicians.

———. 1997. The Urban Health Penalty. American College of Physicians On-Line Position Paper. www.acponline.org/ppvl/policies/e000246.html (accessed September 15, 2008).

Andrulis, D. P., and N. J. Goodman. 1999. *The Social and Health Landscape of Urban and Suburban America.* Chicago: AHA Press.

Andrulis, D. P., and Y. Shaw-Taylor. 1996. The social and health characteristics of California cities. *Health Affairs* 15(1): 131–42.

Ansari, Z. 2007. The concept and usefulness of ambulatory care–sensitive conditions as indicators of quality and access to primary health care. *Australian Journal of Primary Health* 13(3).

Artaud-Wild, S. M., S. L. Connor, G. Sexton, and W. E. Connor. 1993. Lipids/atherosclerosis/arteries: Differences in coronary mortality can be explained by differences in cholesterol and saturated fat intakes in 40 countries but not in France and Finland; A paradox. *Circulation* 88(6): 2771–79.

Ashford, D. E. 1980. *Policy and Politics in Britain: The Limits of Consensus.* Philadelphia: Temple University Press.

Ayanian, J. Z., and A. M. Epstein. 1991. Differences in the use of procedures between men and women hospitalized for coronary heart disease. *New England Journal of Medicine* 325:221–25.

Ayanian, J. Z., I. S. Udvarhelyi, C. A. Gatsonis, C. L. Pashos, and A. M. Epstein. 1993. Racial differences in the use of revascularization procedures after coronary angiography. *Journal of the American Medical Association* 269: 2642–46.

Babazono, A., and A. L. Hillman. 1994. A comparison of international health outcomes and health care spending. *International Journal of Technology Assessment in Health Care* 10(3): 376–81.

Backus, L., M. Moron, P. Baccheti, L. C. Baker, and A. B. Bindman. 2002. Effect of managed care on preventable hospitalization rates in California. *Medical Care* 40(4): 315–24.

Baily, M., and A. M. Garber. 1997. Health care productivity. *Brookings Papers on Economic Activity: Microeconomics* 28:143–2002.

Baldwin, C. 2005. Mayor of London: Access to primary care report—Tower Hamlets PCT given praise for progress. Press Release. Tower Hamlets Primary Care Trust, January 6.

Banks, J., M. Marmot, Z. Oldfield, and J. Smith. 2006. Disease and disadvantage in the United States and England. *Journal of the American Medical Association* 295:2037–45.

Bardsley, M. 1999. *Health in Europe's Capitals.* Project Megépoles. London: Directorate of Public Health, East London, and the City Health Authority.

Barrett-Connor, E. 1997. Sex differences in coronary heart disease: Why are women so superior? The 1995 Ancel Keys lecture. *Circulation* 95:252–64.

Bell, M. R., D. R. Holmes, Jr., P. B. Berger, et al. 1993. The changing in-hospital mortality of women undergoing percutaneous transluminal coronary angioplasty. *Journal of the American Medical Association* 269:2091–95.

Ben-Shlomo, Y., and N. Chaturvedi. 1995. Accessing equity in access to health care provision in the UK: Does where you live affect your chances of getting a coronary artery bypass graft? *Journal of Epidemiology and Community Health* 49:200–204.

Bergelson, B. A., and C. L. Tommaso. 1995. Gender differences in clinical evaluation and triage in coronary artery disease. *Chest* 108:1510–13.

Berk, M. L., C. L. Schur, and J. C. Cantor. 1995. Ability to obtain health care: Recent estimates from the Robert Wood Johnson Foundation National Access to Care Survey. *Health Affairs* 14(3): 139–46.

Berry, B. 1961. *Central Place Studies*. Philadelphia: Regional Science Research Institute.

Berwick, D. 2005. My right knee. *Annals of Internal Medicine* 142:121–25.

Bickell, N. A., K. S. Pieper, K. L. Lee, et al. 1992. Referral patterns for coronary artery disease treatment: Gender bias or good clinical judgment? *Annals of Internal Medicine* 116:791–97.

Billings, J. 2004. Using Administrative Data to Monitor Access, Identify Disparities, and Assess Performance of the Safety Net. Agency for Healthcare Quality Research website. www.ahrq.gov/data/safetynet/billings.htm.

Billings, J., G. M. Anderson, and L. S. Newman. 1996. Recent findings on preventable hospitalizations. *Health Affairs* 15(3): 239–49.

Billings, J., and R. M. Weinick. 2003. *Monitoring the Health Care Safety Net, Book I: A Data Book for Metropolitan Areas*. Washington, DC: Agency for Healthcare Research and Quality.

Billings, J., L. Beitel, J. Lukomnik, T. S. Carey, A. E. Blank, and L. Newman. 1993. Impact of socioeconomic status on hospital use in New York City. *Health Affairs* 12(1): 162–73.

Black, N., S. Langham, C. Coshall, and J. Parker. 1996. Impact of the 1991 NHS reforms on the availability and use of coronary revascularisation in the UK (1987-1995). *Heart* 76(4S): 1–31

Blendon, R., R. Leitman, K. Morrison, and K. Donelan. 1990. Satisfaction with health systems in ten nations. *Health Affairs* 9(2): 185–92.

Blustein, J. 1993. High technology cardiac procedures: The impact of service availability on service use in New York State. *Journal of the American Medical Association* 270:344–49.

Blustein, J., K. Hanson, and S. Shea. 1998. Preventable hospitalizations and socioeconomic status. *Health Affairs* 17(2): 177–89.

BMJ (*British Medical Journal*). 2000. Effect of NHS breast screening programme on mortality from breast cancer in England and Wales, 1990-8: Comparison of observed with predicted mortality. *British Medical Journal* 321:665–69.

Body-Gendrot, S. 1996. Paris: A "soft" global city? *New Community* 22(4): 619–35.

Bots, M. L., and D. E. Grobbee. 1996. Decline of coronary heart disease mortality in the Netherlands from 1978 to1985: Contribution of medical care and changes over time in presence of major cardiovascular risk factors. *Journal of Cardiovascular Risk* 3(3): 271–76.

Bridgman, R. F. 1962. *L'Hôpital et la Cité*. Paris: Editions du Cosmos, Encyclopépie Hospitalière.

Brown, A. D., M. J. Goldacre, and N. Hicks. 2001. Hospitalization for ambulatory-care sensitive conditions: A method for comparing access and quality studies using routinely collected statistics. *Canadian Journal of Public Health* 92: 155–59.

Brown, E. R., R. Wyn, and S. Teleki. 2000. *Disparities in Health Insurance and Access to Care for Residents across U.S. Cities*. New York and Los Angeles: The Commonwealth Fund and UCLA Center for Health Policy Research, August.

Brown, L. D. 1998. Exceptionalism as the rule? U.S. health policy innovation and cross-national learning. *Journal of Health Politics, Policy and Law* 23(1): 35–51.

———. 2003. Comparing health systems in four countries: Lessons for the United States. *American Journal of Public Health* 93(1): 52–56.

Brown, L. D., and M. Sparer. 2003. Poor program's progress: The unanticipated politics of Medicaid policy. *Health Affairs* 22(1): 31.

Buck, D., A. Eastwood, and P. C. Smith. 1999. Can we measure the social importance of health care? *International Journal of Technology Assessment in Health Care* 15:89–107.

Bunker, J. P., H. S. Frazier, and F. Mosteller. 1994. Improving health: Measuring effects of medical care. *Milbank Memorial Fund Quarterly* 72:225–58.

Burke, G. L., S. A. Edlavitch, and R. S. Crow. 1989. The effects of diagnostic criteria on trends in coronary heart disease morbidity: The Minnesota Heart Survey. *Journal of Clinical Epidemiology* 42:17–24.

Cadot, E., V. R. Rodwin, and A. Spira. 2007. In the heat of summer: Lessons from heat waves in Paris. *Journal of Urban Health* 84(4): 466–68.

Camden Primary Care Trust. 2007. Camden PCT Information Briefing. Health Scrutiny Meeting, July 17.

Campbell, J. L., J. Ramsay, J. Green, and K. Harvey. 2005. Forty-eight-hour access to primary care: Practice factors predicting patients' perceptions. *Family Practice* 22:266–68.

Campbell, R. J., A. M. Ramirez, K. Perez, and R. G. Roetzheim. 2003. Cervical cancer rates and the supply of primary care physicians in Florida. *Family Medicine* 35:60–64.

Cantor, J., D. Belloff, C. Schoen, S. How, and D. McCarthy. 2007. *State Scorecard on Health System Performance: Chartpack.* New York: Commonwealth Fund.

Capewell, S., R. Beaglehole, M. Seddon, and J. J. McMurrey. 2000. Explanation for the decline in coronary heart disease mortality in Auckland, New Zealand, between 1982 and 1993. *Circulation* 102:1511–16.

Capewell, S., C. E. Morrison, and J. J. McMurrey. 1999. Contribution of modern cardiovascular treatment and risk factor changes to the decline in coronary heart disease mortality in Scotland between 1975 and 1994. *Heart* 81:380–86.

Carlisle, D. M., B. D. Leake, and M. E. Shapiro. 1997. Racial and ethnic disparities in the use of cardiovascular procedures: Associations with type of health insurance. *American Journal of Public Health* 87:263–67.

Casanova, C., and B. Starfield. 1995. Hospitalizations of children and access to primary care: A cross-national comparison. *International Journal of Health Services* 25(2): 283–94.

Cavelaars, A. E., A. E. Kunst, and J. P. Mackenbach. 1997. Socioeconomic differences in risk factors for morbidity and mortality in the European community: An international comparison. *Journal of Health Psychology* 2:353–72.

Chaix, B., P. J. Veugelers, P.-Y. Boëlle, and P. Chauvin. 2005. Access to general practitioner services: The disabled elderly lag behind in underserved areas. *European Journal of Public Health* 15(3): 282–87.

Charlton, J. R. H., R. M. Hartley, R. Silver, and W. W. Holland. 1986. Geographical variation in mortality from conditions amenable to medical intervention in England and Wales. *Lancet* 1:199–202.

Chassin, M. R. 1993. Explaining geographic variations: The enthusiasm hypothesis. *Medical Care* 31 (Suppl. 5): YS37–44.

Chassin, M. R., R. W. Galvin, and the National Roundtable on Healthcare Quality. 1998. The urgent need to improve health care quality: The National Institute of Medicine Roundtable on Health Care Quality. *Journal of the American Medical Association* 280(11): 1000–1005.

Chernichovsky, D. 1995. Health system reforms in industrialized economies: An emerging paradigm. *Milbank Quarterly* 73(3): 339–72.

Chernichovsky, D. 2002. Pluralism, choice, and the state in the emerging paradigm in health systems. *Milbank Quarterly* 80(1): 5–40.

Cleary, P. D., D. Mechanic, and J. R. Greenley. 1982. Sex differences in medical care utilization: An empirical investigation. *Journal of Health Social Behavior* 23:106–19.

Clinton, W. J. 1998. Address Before a Joint Session of the Congress on the State of the Union. *Weekly Compilation of Presidential Documents.* Washington, DC: Government Printing Office.

Coburn, J. 2004. Confronting the challenges in reconnecting urban planning and public health. *American Journal of Public Health* 94(4): 541–46.

Cochrane, A. L., A. S. St. Leger, and F. Moore. 1978. Health service "input" and mortality "output" in developed countries. *Journal of Epidemiology and Community Health* 32:200–205.

Cohen, D. A., K. Mason, A. Bedimo, et al. 2003. Neighborhood physical conditions and health. *American Journal of Public Health* 93(3): 467–71.

Commission des comptes de la sécurité sociale. 2002. *Les comptes de la sécurité sociale: Résultats 2002, prévisions 2003*. Paris: Ministère de la santé, de la famille et des personnes handicapées.

Cowley, M. J., M. S. Mulin, S. F. Kelsey, et al. 1985. Sex differences in early and long-term results of coronary angioplasty in NHLBI PTCA registry. *Circulation* 71:90–97.

Coyne, J., and P. Hilsenrath. 2002. The World Health Report, 2000. *American Journal of Public Health* 92(1): 30–33.

Crane, R. 2008. Cities: The Missing Presidential Campaign Issue. Op-Ed at Planetzien: The Urban Planning Network, July 14. www.planetizen.com/node/33850.

Cremieux, P.-Y., P. Ouellette, and C. Pilon. 1999. Health care spending as determinants of health outcomes. *Health Economics* 8:627–39.

Cunningham, P., and J. Hadley. 2004. Expanding care versus expanding coverage: How to improve access to care. *Health Affairs* 23(4): 234–44.

Cutler, D. 2003. A framework for evaluating medical care systems. Chap. 7 in OECD, *A Disease-Based Comparison of Health Systems: What Is Best at What Cost?* Paris: OECD.

Dahl, R. A. 1985. *A Preface to Economic Democracy*. Berkeley and Los Angeles: University of California Press.

Davey Smith, G., C. L. Hart, G. Watt, D. Hole, and V. M. Hawthorne. 1998. Individual social class, area-based deprivation, cardiovascular disease risk factors, and mortality: The Renfrew and Paisley Study. *Journal of Epidemiology and Community Health* 52:339–405.

Davis, K. 2007. Learning from high-performance health care systems around the globe. Invited testimony, Senate Health, Education, Labor, and Pensions Committee, *Hearing on Health Care Coverage and Access: Challenges and Opportunities*, January 10. Commonwealth Fund Publication no. 996.

De Kervasdoue, J., J. Kimberly, and V. Rodwin, eds. 1984. *The End of an Illusion: The Future of Health Policy in Western Industrialized Nations*. Berkeley and Los Angeles: University of California Press.

Dobson, F. 1999. Modernizing Britain's national health service. *Health Affairs* 18(3): 40–41.

Dreier, P., J. Mollenkopf, and T. Swanstrom. 2004. *Place Matters: Metropolitics for the Twenty-First Century.* Lawrence: University Press of Kansas.

Duffy, J. 1974. *A History of Public Health in New York City.* New York: Russell Sage.

Dupeyroux, J. J. 1996. *Securité Sociale.* Paris: Dalloz.

Elkin, S. L. 1987. *City and Regime in the American Republic.* Chicago: University of Chicago Press.

Ellen, I., T. Mijanovich, and K. Dillman. 2001. Neighborhood effects on health: Exploring the links and assessing the evidence. *Journal of Urban Affairs* 23:391–408.

Enthoven, A., and R. Kronick. 1989. A consumer-choice health plan for the 1990s: Universal health insurance in a system designed to promote quality and economy. *New England Journal of Medicine* 320:29–37, 94–101.

Ettelt, S., E. N. Nicholas Mays, S. Thomson, M. McKee, and the International Healthcare Comparisons Network. 2006. *Health Care outside Hospital: Accessing Generalist and Specialist Care in Eight Countries.* Policy Brief. World Health Organization on behalf of the European Observatory on Health Systems and Policies.

Evandrou, M. 2006. Inequalities amongst older people in London: The challenge of diversity. Chap. 9 in Rodwin and Gusmano, *Growing Older in World Cities.*

Field, M., and H. Shapiro, eds. 1993. *Employment and Health Benefits: A Connection at Risk.* Washington, DC: Institute of Medicine.

Fitzpatrick, A. L., N. R. Powe, L. S. Cooper, D. G. Ives, and J. A. Robbins. 2004. Barriers to health care access among the elderly and who perceives them. *American Journal of Public Health* 94(10): 1788–94.

Flora, P., and P. Heidenheimer. 1981. *The Development of Welfare States in Europe and America.* New Brunswick, NJ: Transaction Books.

Florida, R. 2005. *Cities and the Creative Class.* New York: Routledge.

Fogel, R. W. 2000. The extension of life in the twentieth century and its implications for social policy in the twenty-first century. *Population and Development Review* 26 (Supplement: Population and Economic Change in East Asia): 291–317.

Fossett, J., and J. Perloff. 1995. The "new" health reform and access to care: The problem of the inner city. Washington, DC: Kaiser Commission on the Future of Medicaid, December.

Friedmann, J. 1986. The world city hypothesis. *Development and Change* 17:69–84.

Geronimus, A. T. 1996. What teen mothers know. *Human Nature* 7(4): 323–52.

Ginsberg, E., H. S. Berliner, and M. Ostow. 1993. *Changing U.S. Health Care: A Study of Four Metropolitan Areas.* Sudbury, MA: Westview Press.

Ginsberg, P. 1996. The RWJF Community Snapshots study: Introduction and overview. *Health Affairs* 15(2): 7–20.

Glied, S., and S. E. Little. 2003. The uninsured and the benefits of medical progress. *Health Affairs* 22(4): 210.

Goodman, J. C., G. Musgrave, and D. Herrick. 2004. *Lives at Risk: Single-Payer National Health Insurance around the World.* Lanham, MD: Rowman & Littlefield.

Golino, A., A. Panza, G. Janelli, et al. 1991. Myocardial revascularization in women. *Texas Heart Institute Journal* 18:194–98.

Gottschalk, M. 2007. Back to the future? Health benefits, organized labor, and universal health care. *Journal of Health Politics, Policy and Law* 32(6): 923–70

Gravelle, H. S., and M. E. Backhouse. 1987. International cross-section analysis of the determination of mortality. *Social Science and Medicine* 25(5): 427–41.

Greene, W. H. 2000. *Econometric Analysis.* 4th ed. Upper Saddle River, NJ: Prentice-Hall.

Greer, A. L., and S. A. Greer. 1983. *Cities and Sickness: Health Care in Urban America.* Thousand Oaks, CA: Sage Publications.

Gregory, P. M., E. S. Malka, J. B. Kostis, et al. 2000. Impact of geographic proximity to cardiac revascularization services on service utilization. *Medical Care* 38:45–57.

Grogan, C. M., and M. K. Gusmano. 2007. *Healthy Voices, Unhealthy Silence.* Washington, DC: Georgetown University Press.

Grumbach, K., G. M. Anderson, H. S. Luft, L. L. Roos, and R. Brook. 1995. Regionalization of cardiac surgery in the United States and Canada: Geographic access, choice, and outcomes. *Journal of the American Medical Association* 274:1282–88.

Gurr, T., and D. King. 1987. *The State and the City.* London: Macmillan.

Gusmano, M. K. 2008. History of geriatric healthcare in America: How does the US compare to other nations in the care of its elderly? Paper presented at Metropolitan Area Geriatrics Society Meeting, "State of Health Care for Older Americans," New York Academy of Medicine, New York, April 16, 2008.

Gusmano, M. K., and J.-P. Michel. 2009. Life course vaccination and healthy aging. *Aging Clinical and Experimental Research* 21(3): 258–63.

Gusmano, M. K., and V. G. Rodwin. 2005. Health services research and the city. In D. Vlahov and S. Galea, eds., *Handbook of Urban Health.* New York: Springer.

Gusmano, M. K., and V. G. Rodwin. 2006. Growing older in world cities: Themes, interpretations, and future research. Chap. 23 in Rodwin and Gusmano, *Growing Older in World Cities.*

Gusmano, M. K., V. G. Rodwin, and M. Cantor. 2007. Old and poor in New York City. Policy Brief, International Longevity Center–USA. New York, February.

Gusmano, M. K., V. G. Rodwin, D. Weisz, and D. Das. 2007. A new approach to the comparative analysis of health systems: Invasive treatment for heart disease in the U.S., France, and their two world cities. *Health Economics, Policy and Law* 2:73–92.

Hadley, J., E. P. Steinberg, and J. Feder. 1991. Comparison of uninsured and privately insured hospital patients: Condition on admission, resource use, and outcome. *Journal of the American Medical Association* 265(3): 374–79.

Hakama, M., E. Pukkala, K. V. Heikkilä, et al. 1997. Effectiveness of the public health policy for breast cancer screening in Finland: Population-based cohort study. *British Medical Journal* 314:864–67.

Hall, P. 1998. *Cities in Civilization*. New York: Pantheon.

Healy, B. 1991. The Yentl syndrome. Editorial. *New England Journal of Medicine* 325:274–76.

Hochman, J. S., J. E. Tamis, T. D. Thompson, et al. 1999. Sex, clinical presentation, and outcome in patients with acute coronary syndromes. *New England Journal of Medicine* 341:226–32.

Holland, W., ed. 1997. *European Community Atlas of Avoidable Death, 1985–1989*. 3rd ed. Oxford: Oxford University Press.

Howard, C. 1993. The hidden side of the American welfare state. *Political Science Quarterly* 108(3): 403–36.

HUD (U.S. Department of Housing and Urban Development). 1999. *The State of the Cities, 1999*. www.huduser.org/publications/polleg/tsoc99/contents.html (accessed August 29, 2009).

———. 2002. *The American Community Survey: Challenges and Opportunities for HUD*. Washington, DC: U.S. Government Printing Office.

Hunink, M. G. M., I. Goldman, A. N. A. Tosteson, et al. 1997. The recent decline in mortality from coronary heart disease, 1980–1990. *Journal of the American Medical Association* 277:535–42.

Hurst, J., and J.-P. Poullier. 1993. Paths to health reform. *OECD Observer*, vol. a.

Hussey, P. S., G. F. Anderson, R. Osborne, et al. 2004. How does the quality of care compare in five countries? *Health Affairs* 23(3): 89–99.

Iezzoni, L. I., A. S. Ash, M. Shwartz, and Y. Mackiernan. 1997. Differences in procedure use, in-hospital mortality, and illness severity by gender for acute myocardial infarction patients: Are answers affected by data source and severity measure? *Medical Care* 35:158–71.

Illich, I. 1976. *Limits to Medicine*. London: Marion Boyars.

International Diabetes Federation. 2006. *Diabetes Atlas*. 3rd ed. Brussels: International Diabetes Federation. www.eatlas.idf.org.

Jacobs, A. K., S. F. Kelsey, M. M. Brooks, et al. 1998. Better outcome for women compared with men undergoing coronary revascularization: A report from the Bypass Angioplasty Revascularization Investigation (BARI). *Circulation* 98:1279–85.

Jacobs, J. 1961. *Death and Life of Great American Cities.* New York: Vintage.

Jones, B. D., and L. W. Bachelor. 1986. *The Sustaining Hand: Community Leadership and Corporate Power.* Lawrence: University of Kansas Press.

Jougla, E., P. Ducimetière, M. H. Bouvier-Colle, and F. Hatton. 1987. Relation entre le niveau de développement du système de soins et le niveau de la mortalité évitable selon les départements français. *Revue d'Epidemiologie et de Sante Publique* 35:365–77.

Judd, D. R., and T. Swanstrom. 1994. *City Politics.* New York: HarperCollins College Publishers.

Kasper, J. D., T. A. Giovannini, and C. Hoffman. 2000. Gaining and losing health insurance: Strengthening the evidence for effects on access to care and health outcomes. *Medical Care Research and Review* 57(3): 298–318.

Khan, S. S., S. Nessim, R. Gray, et al. 1990. Increased mortality of women in coronary artery bypass surgery: Evidence for referral bias. *Annals of Internal Medicine* 112:561–67.

King, L. J. 1984. *Central Place Theory.* Beverly Hills, CA: Sage Publications.

Klein, R. 1997. Learning from others: Shall the last be the first? *Journal of Health Politics, Policy and Law* 22(5): 1267–78.

———. 2001. Estimating the financial requirements of health care: The Wanless report is a pioneering effort—with a few omissions and errors. *British Medical Journal* 323:1318–19.

Klein, R. J., and C. A. Schoenborn. 2001. Age adjustment using the 2000 projected U.S. population. *Healthy People 2010 Statistical Notes,* no. 20 (January).

Koeppel, G. T. 2000. *Water for Gotham: A History.* Princeton: Princeton University Press.

Komaromy, M., N. Lurie, D. Osmond, et al. 1996. Physician practice style and rates of hospitalization for chronic medical conditions. *Medical Care* 34(6): 594–609.

Laditka, J. N., S. B. Laditka, and M. P. Mastanduno. 2003. Hospital utilization for ambulatory care sensitive conditions: Health outcome disparities associated with race and ethnicity. *Social Science and Medicine* 57(8): 1429–41.

Lantz, P. M., J. S. House, J. M. Lepkowski, D. R. Williams, R. P. Mero, and J. Chen. 1998. Socioeconomic factors, health behaviors, and mortality: Results from a nationally representative prospective study of U.S. adults. *Journal of the American Medical Association.* 279:1703–8.

LaVeist, T. A., and Wallace, J. M., Jr. 2000. Health risk and inequitable distribution of liquor stores in African American neighborhood. *Social Science and Medicine* 51:613–17.

Leape, L. L., L. H. Hilborne, R. Bell, C. Kamberg, and R. H. Brook. 1999. Underuse of cardiac procedures: Do women, ethnic minorities, and the uninsured fail to receive needed revascularization? *Annals of Internal Medicine* 130: 183–92.

Leatherman, S., and K. Sutherland. 2008. *The Quest for Quality in the NHS: Refining the NHS Reforms.* London: Nuffield Trust.

Lefèvre, H., E. Jougla, G. Pavillon, and A. Le Toulle. 2004. Disparitiès de mortalité "prématuré" selon le sexe et causes de décès évitables. *Revue Epidemiology Sainte Publique* 52:317–28.

Le Grand, J. 1999. Competition, cooperation, or control? Tales from the British National Health Service. *Health Affairs* 18(3): 27–39.

LePen, C., and V. G. Rodwin. 1996. Le Plan Juppé: Vers un nouveux mode de régulation des soins. *Droit Social* 9(10): 859–62.

Levey, N. N. 2009. Obama signs into law expansion of SCHIP health-care program for children. *Chicago Tribune,* February 5. www.chicagotribune.com/news/nationworld/chi-kids-health-care_thufebo5,0,30310.story.

Lewin, M. E., and S. Altman. 2000. *America's Health Care Safety-Net: Intact but Endangered.* Washington, DC: National Academy Press.

Liff, J. M., W. H. Chow, and R. S. Greenberg. 1991. Rural-urban differences in stage at diagnosis: Possible relationship to cancer screening. *Cancer* 67(5): 1454–59.

Lindblom, C. E. 1977. *Politics and Markets: The World's Political-Economic Systems.* New York: Basic Books.

Linden, E. 1996. The exploding cities of the developing world. *Foreign Affairs* 75(1): 52–65.

Litman, T. J., and L. S. Robins, eds. 1991. *Health Politics and Policy.* 2nd ed. New York: Delmar Publishers.

London Health Commission. 2007. *Health in London.* London: UK Department of Health.

Lucas-Gabrielli, V., P. Pépin, and F. Tonnellier. 2006. The health of older Parisians. Chap. 13 in Rodwin and Gusmano, *Growing Older in World Cities.*

Lynch, J. W., G. A. Kaplan, and J. T. Salonen. 1997. Why do poor people behave poorly? Variation in adult health behaviours and psychosocial characteristics by stage of the socioeconomic lifecourse. *Social Science and Medicine* 44(2): 810–19.

Macinko, J., B. Starfield, and L. Shi. 2003. The contribution of primary care systems to health outcomes within Organization for Economic Cooperation and Development (OECD) countries, 1970-1998. *Health Services Research* 38:831–65.

Mackenbach, J. P. 1996. The contribution of medical care to mortality decline: McKeown revisited. *Journal of Clinical Epidemiology* 49:1207–13.

Mackenbach, J. P., C. W. N. Looman, A. L. Kunst, J. D. I. Habbema, and P. J. van der Maas. 1998. Post-1950 mortality trends and medical care: Gains in life expectancy due to declines in mortality from conditions amenable to medical intervention in the Netherlands. *Social Science and Medicine* 27:889–94.

Mainous, A. G., and F. P. Kohrs. 2005. A comparison of health status between rural and urban adults. *Journal of Community Health* 20(5): 423–31.

Marmor, T. R. 1973. *The Politics of Medicare.* Chicago: Aldine.

Marmor, T., R. Freeman, and K. Okma. 2005. Comparative perspectives and policy learning in the world of health care. *Journal of Comparative Policy Analysis* 7(4): 331–48.

Marmor, T., and J. Mashaw. 2006. Understanding social insurance: Fairness, affordability, and the "modernization" of Social Security and Medicare. Web Exclusive. *Health Affairs* 25 March 21): w114–34. http://content.healthaffairs .org/cgi/content/abstract/hlthaff.25.w114v1

Marshall, M., S. Leatherman, S. Mattke, et al. 2004. *Selecting Indicators for the Quality of Health Promotion, Prevention, and Primary Care at the Health Systems Level in OECD Countries.* OECD Health Technical Papers, no. 16. Paris: OECD.

Mayor of London. 2004. Primary care access in London. Briefing. London, Office of the Mayor, November.

McGlynn, E. 2004. There is no perfect health system. *Health Affairs* 23(3): 100–102.

McKeown T. 1979. *The Role of Medicine: Dream, mirage or nemesis?* Oxford: Blackwell.

McKinlay, J. B., and S. M. McKinlay. 1977. The questionable contribution of medical measures to the decline of mortality in the United States in the twentieth century. *Milbank Memorial Fund Quarterly* 55:405–28.

McKinsey Global Institute. 1996. *Health Care Productivity.* Washington, DC.

Mickleborough, L. L., Y. Takagi, H. Maruyama, et al. 1995. Is sex a factor in determining operative risk for aortocoronary bypass graft surgery? *Circulation* 92 (Suppl. 9): 80–84.

Millman, M., ed. 1993. *Access to Health Care in America.* Washington, DC: National Academy Press.

Mindell, J., E. Klodawski, J. Fitzpatrick, N. Malhotra, M. McKee, and C. Sanderson. 2008. The impact of private-sector provision on equitable utilisation of coronary revascularisation in London. *Heart* (British Cardiac Society) 94(8):1008–11.

Moise, P., and S. Jacobzone. 2003. Population ageing, health expenditure, and treatment: An ARD perspective. Chap. 10 in OECD, *A Disease-Based Comparison of Health Systems: What Is Best at What Cost?* Paris: OECD.

Mollenkopf, J., and M. Castells, eds. 1991. *Dual City: Restructuring New York.* New York: Russell Sage Foundation.

Morone, J. A. 1993. The health care bureaucracy: Small changes, great consequences. *Journal of Health Politics, Policy and Law* 18:3.

Morone, J. A., and A. Dunham. 1985. Slouching towards national health insurance: The new health care politics. *Yale Journal of Regulation* 2(2): 263–91.

Mullan, F. 1998. The "Mona Lisa" of health policy: Primary care at home and abroad. *Health Affairs* 17(2): 118–26.

Muller, C. F. 1990. *Health Care and Gender.* New York: Russell Sage Foundation.

Mumford, L. 1938. *The Culture of Cities.* New York: Harcourt Brace.

National Association of City and County Health Officials. 2007. *Big Cities Health Inventory, 2007: The Health of Urban USA.* www.who.or.jp/2008/urbanh/US _Big_Cities_Healt_Inventory_2007.pdf.

National Health Service and Commission for Racial Equality. 2004. *Race Equality Guide, 2004: A Performance Framework.* London: North Central London Strategic Health Authority.

Navarro, V. 2002. The World Health Report, 2000: Can health care systems be compared using a single measure of performance? *American Journal of Public Health* 92(1): 31–34.

Nestle, M. 1994. Diet and alcohol in heart disease risk: The French paradox. *Contemporary Drug Problems,* Spring, 71–76.

New York City. 2004a. Community Health Survey. Department of Health and Mental Hygiene. www.nyc.gov/html/doh/html/survey/survey.shtml (accessed August 29, 2009).

———. 2004b. *Take Care New York.* Department of Health and Mental Hygiene. www.nyc.gov/html/doh/html/tcny.

———. 2009. Colon Cancer Control Coalition website. Department of Health and Mental Hygiene. www.nyc.gov/html/doh/html/cancer/cancercolon.shtml (accessed August 29, 2009).

Nixon, J., and P. Ulmann. 2006. The relationship between health care expenditure and health outcomes: Evidence and caveats for a causal link. *European Journal of Health Economics* 7(1): 7–18.

Nolte, E., and M. McKee. 2003. Measuring the health of nations: Analysis of mortality amenable to health care. *British Medical Journal* 328: 327–494.

———. 2004. *Does Health Care Save Lives? Avoidable Mortality Revisited.* London: Nuffield Trust.

Northridge, M. E., and E. Sclar. 2003. A joint urban planning and public health framework: Contributions to health impact assessment. *American Journal of Public Health* 93(1): 118–21.

O'Connor, G. T., J. R. Morton, M. J. Diehl, et al. 1993. The Northern New England Cardiovascular Disease Study Group: Differences between men and women in hospital mortality associated with coronary artery bypass graft surgery. *Circulation* 88:2104–10.

OECD. 2000–2006. *OECD Health Data, 2000–2006: Comparative Analysis of 30 Countries.* Paris: OECD.

Oliver, A. 2005. The English National Health Service, 1979–2005. *Health Economics* 14 (Suppl. 1): S75–99.

Oliver, A., A. Healey, and J. Le Grand. 2002. Addressing health inequalities. *Lancet* 360:565–67.

Olshansky, S., D. J. Passaro, R. C. Hershow, et al. 2005. A potential decline in life expectancy in the United States in the 21st century. *New England Journal of Medicine* 352:1138–45.

Or, Z. 2000. Determinants of health outcomes in industrialised countries: A pooled, cross-country, time-series analysis. *OECD Economic Studies* 30: 53–77.

———. 2001. *Exploring the effects of health care on mortality across OECD countries: Labour Market and Social Policy.* Occasional Papers No. 46. Paris: OECD.

Orr, M. 1992. Urban regimes and human capital policies: A study of Baltimore. *Journal of Urban Affairs* 14(2): 173–87.

Oster, A., and A. B. Bindman. 2003. Emergency department visits for ambulatory care sensitive conditions: Insights into preventable hospitalizations. *Medical Care* 41(2): 198–207.

Paine, L. H. W., ed. 1978. *Health Care in Big Cities.* New York: St. Martin's Press.

Pappas, G., W. C. Hadden, L. J. Kozak, and G. F. Fisher. 1997. Potentially avoidable hospitalizations: Inequalities in rates between US socioeconomic groups. *American Journal of Public Health* 87(5): 811–16.

Parchman, M. L., and S. Culler. 1994. Primary care physicians and avoidable hospitalizations. *Journal of Family Practice* 39(2): 123–28.

Pashos, C. L., J. P. Newhouse, and B. J. McNeil. 1993. Temporal changes in the care and outcomes of elderly patients with acute myocardial infarction, 1987 through 1990. *Journal of the American Medical Association* 270:1832–36.

Perrin, J. M., C. J. Homer, D. M. Berwick, A. D. Woolf, J. L. Freeman, and J. E. Wennberg. 1990. Variations in rates of hospitalization of children in three urban communities. *New England Journal of Medicine* 322(3): 206–7.

Peterson, P. E. 1981. *City Limits*. Chicago: University of Chicago Press.

Peto, J., C. Gilham, O. Fletcher, and F. E Matthews. 2004. The cervical cancer epidemic that screening has prevented in the UK. *Lancet* 364:249–56.

Philbin, E. F., P. A. McCullough, T. G. DiSalvo, G. W. Dec, P. L. Jenkins, and W. D. Weaver. 2001. Underuse of invasive procedures among Medicaid patients with acute myocardial infarction. *American Journal of Public Health* 91:1082–88.

Pilote, L., R. M. Califf, S. Sapp, et al. 1995. Regional variation across the United States in the management of acute myocardial infarction. *New England Journal of Medicine* 333:565–72.

Poikolainen, K., and J. Eskola. 1986. Mortality from causes amenable to health services intervention. *Lancet* 1:199–202.

Politzer, R., D. Harris, M. Gaston, et al. 1991. Primary care physician supply and the medically underserved. *Journal of the American Medical Association* 266:104–9.

Popescu, I., M. S. Vaughan-Sarrazin, and G. E. Rosenthal. 2007. Differences in mortality and use of revascularization in black and white patients with acute MI admitted to hospitals with and without revascularization services. *Journal of the American Medical Association* 297:2489–95.

Propper, C., and R. Upward. 1992. Need, equity and the NHS: The distribution of health care expenditure, 1974-87. *Fiscal Studies* 13(2): 1–21.

Rahimtoola, S. H., A. J. Bennett, G. L. Grunkmeier, et al. 1993. Survival at 15 to 18 years after coronary bypass surgery for angina in women. *Circulation* 88:II71–78.

Raine, R. A., N. A. Black, T. J. Bowker, and D. A. Wood. 2002. Gender differences in the management and outcome of patients with acute coronary artery disease. *Journal of Epidemiology and Community Health* 56:791–97.

Reidpath, D., P. A. Allotey, A. Kouame, and R. A. Cummins. 2003. Measuring health in a vacuum: Examining the disability weight of the DALE. *Health Policy and Planning* 18(4): 351.

Reinhardt, U., P. Hussey, and G. Anderson. 1999. Cross-national comparisons of health systems using OECD data. *Health Affairs* 21:169–81.

Renaud, S., and R. Gueguen. 1998. The French paradox and wine drinking. *Novartis Foundation Symposium* 216:208–17.

Reschovsky, J. D., B. C. Strunk, and P. Ginsburg. 2006. Why employer-sponsored coverage changed, 1997-2003. *Health Affairs* 25(3): 774–82.

Richardson, J., J. Wildman, and I. K. Robertson. 2003. A critique of the World Health Organisation's evaluation of health system performance. *Health Economics* 12(5): 355–66.

Rivett, G. 1986. *Development of the London Hospital System, 1823-1982.* London: King's Fund.

Rock, M. 2000. Discounted lives? Weighing disability when measuring health and ruling on "compassionate" murder. *Social Science and Medicine* 51(3): 407.

Rodwin, V. G. 1984. *The Health Planning Predicament: France, Quebec, England, and the United States.* Berkeley and Los Angeles: University of California Press.

———. 2003. The French health system under French National Health Insurance: Lessons for health reform in the United States. *American Journal of Public Health* 93(1): 31–37.

Rodwin, V. G., C. Brecher, D. Jolly, and R. J. Baxter, eds. 1992. *Public Hospital Systems in New York City and Paris.* New York: New York University Press.

Rodwin, V. G., and M. K. Gusmano. 2002. The World Cities Project: Rationale, organization, and design for comparison of megacity health systems. *Journal of Urban Health* 79(4): 445–63.

———, eds. 2006a. *Growing Older in World Cities: New York, London, Paris, and Tokyo.* Nashville: Vanderbilt University Press.

———. 2006b. How can we compare New York, London, Paris, and Tokyo? Defining spatial units of analysis. Chap. 2 in Rodwin and Gusmano, *Growing Older in World Cities.*

Rodwin, V. G., and C. LePen. 2005. French health care reform: The birth of state-led managed care. *New England Journal of Medicine* 351(22): 2259–61.

Rodwin, V. G., and L. G. Neuberg. 2005. Infant mortality and income in four world cities: New York, London, Paris, and Tokyo. *American Journal of Public Health* 98:86–90.

Rosenfield, A., and E. Figdor. 2001. Where is the M in MTCT? The broader issues in mother-to-child transmission of HIV. *American Journal of Public Health* 91(5): 703–4.

Roos, N. P., and C. Mustard. 1997. Variation in health and health care use by socioeconomic status in Winnipeg, Canada: Does the system work well? Yes and no. *Milbank Quarterly* 75:89–111.

Rosenfield, A., and D. Maine. 1985. Maternal mortality—a neglected tragedy: Where is the M in MCH? *Lancet* 2:83–85.

Rosenfield, A., C. J. Min, and L. P. Freedman. 2007. Making motherhood safe in developing countries. *New England Journal of Medicine* 356(14): 1395–96.

Rosner, D. 1982. *A Once Charitable Enterprise: Hospitals and Health Care in Brooklyn and New York, 1885-1915.* Cambridge: Cambridge University Press.

Rouleau, J. L., L. A. Moye, M. A. Pfeffer, et al. 1993. A comparison of management patterns after acute myocardial infarction in Canada and the United States. *New England Journal of Medicine* 328:779–84.

Rutstein, D. D., W. Berenberg, T. C. Chalmers, C. G. Child, A. P. Fishman, and E. B. Perrin. 1976. Measuring the quality of health care. *New England Journal of Medicine* 294:582–88.

Saha, S., G. D. Stettin, and R. F. Redberg. 1999. Gender and willingness to undergo invasive cardiac procedures. *Journal of General Internal Medicine* 14: 122–25.

Sanderson, C., and J. Dixon. 2000. Conditions for which onset or hospital admission is potentially preventable by timely and effective ambulatory care. *Journal of Health Services Research and Policy* 5(4): 222–30.

Sandman, D., C. Schoen, and C. Des Roches. 1998. *The Commonwealth Fund Survey of Health Care in New York City.* New York: Commonwealth Fund, February.

Sante, M., C. Allemani, F. Berrino, et al. 2003. Breast carcinoma survival in Europe and the United States: A population-based study. *Cancer* 100(4): 715–22.

Sassen, S. 2001. *The Global City: New York, London, Tokyo.* 2nd ed. Princeton: Princeton University Press.

Saver, B. 1996. *Access to Ambulatory Care by the Indigent.* Final Report, AHCPR Small Grant No. 1 RO3 HS07253. September. NTIS PB97-134456.

Savitch, H. V., and P. Kantor. 2002. *Cities in the International Marketplace: The Political Economy of Urban Development in North America and Western Europe.* Princeton: Princeton University Press.

Schoen, C., K. Davis, S. K. H. How, and S. C. Schoenbaum. 2006. U.S. health system performance: A national scorecard. Web Exclusive. *Health Affairs.* DOI:10.1377/hlthaff.25.w457.

Schoen, C., R. Osborn, P. T. Huynh, et al. 2006. On the front lines of care: Primary care doctors' office systems, experiences, and views in seven countries. Web Exclusive. *Health Affairs.* DOI:10.1377/hlthaff.25.w555.

Schreyögg, J., T. Stargardt, O. Tiemann, and R. Busse. 2006. Methods to determine reimbursement rates for diagnosis-related groups (DRG): A comparison of nine European countries. *Health Care Management Science* 9:215–23.

Schulz, A. J., D. R. Williams, B. A. Israel, and L. B. Lempert. 2002. Racial and spatial relations as fundamental determinants of health in Detroit. *Milbank Quarterly* 80(4): 677–707.

Senior, R. 2006. To revascularize or not to revascularize: A dilemma in heart failure. *Canadian Medical Association Journal* 175(4). DOI:10.1503/cmaj.060882.

Sheifer, S. E., J. J. Escarce, and K. A. Schulman. 2000. Race and sex differences in the management of coronary artery disease. *American Heart Journal* 139:848–57.

Shi, L. 1992. The relationship between primary care and life chances. *Journal of Health Care for the Poor and Underserved* 3:321–35.

———. 1994. Primary care, specialty care, and life chances. *International Journal of Health Services* 24:431–58.

Shi, L., J. Macinko, B. Starfield, J. Wulu, J. Regan, and R. Politzer. 2003. The relationship between primary care, income inequality, and mortality in the United States, 1980–1995. *Journal of the American Board of Family Practice* 16:412–22.

Shi, L., and B. Starfield. 2000. Primary care, income inequality, and self-rated health in the United States: A mixed-level analysis. *International Journal of Health Services* 30:541–55.

Shi, L., B. Starfield, B. P. Kennedy, and I. Kawachi. 1999. Income inequality, primary care, and health indicators. *Journal of Family Practice* 48:275–84.

Smee, C. 2000. Reconsidering the role of competition in health care markets: United Kingdom. *Journal of Health Politics, Policy and Law* 25(5): 945–51.

Socolar, S., V. W. Sidel, A. R. de Arellano, and F. Goldsmith. 2001. *Strengthening New York City's Public Health Infrastructure*. New York: Public Health Association of New York City. www.phanyc.org/publications (accessed June 29, 2009).

Sparer, M. 2007. Medicaid Federalism and the Politics of National Health Insurance. Paper presented at the American Political Science Association Meeting, Chicago, August 17.

Starfield, B., L. Shi, and J. Macinko. 2005. Contribution of primary care to health systems and health. *Milbank Quarterly* 83(3): 457–502.

Starr, P. 1982. *The Social Transformation of American Medicine*. New York: Basic Books.

Steingart, R. M., M. Packer, P. Hamm, et al. 1991. Sex differences in the management of coronary artery disease. *New England Journal of Medicine* 325:226–30.

Stevens, S. 2004. Reform strategies for the English NHS. *Health Affairs* 23(3): 37–44.

Stone, C. N. 1989. *Regime Politics: Governing Atlanta, 1946–1988*. Kansas: University Press of Kansas.

Stuckler, D. 2008. Population causes and consequences of leading chronic diseases: A comparative analysis of prevailing explanations. *Milbank Quarterly* 86(2): 273–326.

Suhrcke, M., M. McKee, D. Stuckler, R. Sauto Arce, S. Tsolova, and J. Mortensen. 2006. The contribution of health to the economy in the European Union. *Public Health* 120(11): 994–1001.

Tabar, L., G. Fagerberg, S. W. Duffy, et al. 1992. Update of the Swedish two-county program of mammographic screening for breast cancer. *Radiologic Clinics of North America* 30:187–210.

Technological Change in Health Care Research Network. 2001. Technological change around the world: Evidence from heart attack care. *Health Affairs* 20(3): 25–42.

Thorpe, K., and D. Howard. 2006. The rise in spending among Medicare beneficiaries: The role of chronic disease prevalence and changes in treatment intensity. *Health Affairs* 25:w378–w388. http://content.healthaffairs.org/cgi/reprint/25/5/w378.

Tobias, M., and G. Jackson. 2001. Avoidable mortality in New Zealand, 1981-97. *Australian and New Zealand Journal of Public Health* 25:12–20.

Tobier, M. 2006. Growing old in the city that never sleeps. Chap. 3 in Rodwin and Gusmano, *Growing Older in World Cities*.

Treurniet, H. F., H. C. Boshuizen, and P. P. M. Harteloh. 2004. Avoidable mortality in Europe (1980–1997): A comparison of trends. *Journal of Epidemiology and Community Health* 58:290–95.

Treurniet, H. F., C. W. Looman, P. J. van der Maas, and J. P. Mackenbach. 1999. Variations in "avoidable" mortality: A reflection of variations in incidence? *International Journal of Epidemiology* 28:225–32.

Tunstall-Pedoe, H. 1988. Autres pays, autres moeurs. Editorial. *British Medical Journal* 297:1559–60.

Tunstall-Pedoe, H., K. Kuulasmaa, P. Amouyel, D. Arveiler, A. M. Rajakangas, and A. Pajak. 1994. Myocardial infarction and coronary deaths in the World Health Organization Monica Project: Registration procedures, event rates, and case-fatality rates in 38 populations from 21 countries in four continents. *Circulation* 90(1): 583–612.

Unal, B., J. A. Critchley, and S. Capewell. 2004. Explaining the decline in coronary heart disease mortality in England and Wales between 1981 and 2000. *Circulation* 109:1101–7.

———. 2005. Modelling the decline in coronary heart disease deaths in England and Wales, 1981-2000: Comparing contributions from primary prevention and secondary prevention. *British Medical Journal* DOI:10.1136/bmj.38561. 633345.8F (published August 17, 2005).

U.K. Department of Health. 1989. *Working for Patients*. White Paper. London: Her Majesty's Stationery Office.

———. 2000. The NHS Plan: A plan for investment, a plan for reform. Command Paper, July 1.

United Nations. 2008. *State of the World's Cities, 2008/2009: Harmonious Cities*. United Nations Human Settlements Programme (UN-HABITAT). www.unhabitat.org/pmss.

U.S. Preventive Services Task Force. 1996. *Guide to Clinical Preventative Services*. 2nd ed. Baltimore: Williams & Wilkins.

Vaccarino, V., J. L. Abramson, E. Veledar, and W. S. Weintraub. 2002. Sex differences in hospital mortality after coronary bypass surgery: Evidence for a higher mortality in younger women. *Circulation* 105:1176–81.

Vlahov, D., and S. Gallea. 2002. Urbanization, urbanicity, and health. *Journal of Urban History* 79, Supplement 1 (4): S1–11.

Vogel, R. L., and R. J. Ackermann. 1998. Is primary care physician supply correlated with health outcomes? *International Journal of Health Services* 28:183–96.

Warnes, A. 2006. Aging, health, and social services in London. Chap. 8 in Rodwin and Gusmano, *Growing Older in World Cities*.

Weissman, J. S., C. Gatsonis, and A. M. Epstein. 1992. Rates of avoidable hospitalization by insurance status in Massachusetts and Maryland. *Journal of the American Medical Association* 268(17): 2388–94.

Weisz, D., and M. K. Gusmano. 2006. The health of older New Yorkers. Chap. 4 in Rodwin and Gusmano, *Growing Older in World Cities*.

Weisz, D., M. K. Gusmano, and V. G. Rodwin. 2004. Gender and the treatment of heart disease in the United States, France, and England: A comparative population-based view of a clinical phenomenon. *Gender Medicine* 1:29–40.

Wennberg, J. E. 1987. Population illness rates do not explain population hospitalization rates. *Medical Care* 25(4): 354–59.

Wennberg, J. E., B. A. Barnes, and M. Zubkoff. 1982. Professional uncertainty and the problem of supplier-induced demand. *Social Science and Medicine* 16:811–24.

Wennberg, J. E., J. L. Freeman, and W. J. Culp. 1987. Are hospital services rationed in New Haven or over-utilised in Boston? *Lancet* 1:1185–89.

Wennberg, J. E., and A. Gittlesohn. 1973. Small-area variations in health care delivery. *Science* 182:1102–8.

White, J. 1995. *Competing Solutions: American Health Care Proposals and International Experiences*. Washington, DC: Brookings Institution Press.

———. 1998. Old wine, cracked bottle? Tokyo, Paris, and the global city hypothesis. *Urban Affairs Review* 33(4): 451–77.

———. 2007. Markets and medical care: The United States, 1993–2005. *Milbank Quarterly* 85(3): 395–448.

Wilensky, H. L. 1975. *The Welfare State and Equality: Structural and Ideological Roots of Public Expenditures*. Berkeley and Los Angeles: University of California Press.

Wilkinson, R., and M. Marmot. 2003. *Social Determinants of Health: The Solid Facts*. 2nd ed. Denmark: World Health Organization. www.euro.who.int/document/e81384.pdf (accessed November 16, 2006).

Williams, A. 2001. Science or marketing at WHO? A commentary on "World Health 2000." *Health Economics* 10:93–100.

Williams, B., P. Whatmough, J. McGill, and L. Rushton. 2000. Private funding of elective hospital treatment in England and Wales, 1997–8: National survey. *British Medical Journal* 320:904–5.

WHO (World Health Organization). 2000. *The World Health Report, 2000—Health Systems: Improving Performance.* Geneva: World Health Organization.

———. 2006. *World Health Statistics Report, 2006.* www.who.int/whosis/whostat2006_erratareduce.pdf (accessed August 29, 2009).

World Bank. 1993. *World Development Report, 1993: Investing in Health.* New York: Oxford University Press. Available online at www-wds.worldbank.org.

INDEX

Access to care, viii; consequences of limited, 7, 19; different levels of, x
Acute myocardial infarction (AMI), 16, 18, 19, 95–96, 122; diagnostic criteria for, 97; as proxy for burden of IHD, 97–98, and use of revascularization, 101–103
Age-adjustment, 83–84, 93
Agency for Healthcare Research and Quality (AHRQ), 74
American Heart Association, 58, 96
Appendicitis, 17, 82, 83
Assistance Publique–Hôpitaux de Paris (AP-HP), 44–46
Asthma, 17, 74, 83
Australia, 12
Avoidable hospital conditions (AHCs), viii, 17, 73, 75, 94, 108, 122; as accepted measure of access, 74, 80–82; definition of, 83–84; and French primary care system, 79–80; and insurance status, 85–86; and prevalence of disease, 90; and safety-net institutions, 91–92
Avoidable mortality, viii, ix, 15, 56; and data limitations, 60; definition of, 61–62; and socioeconomic status, 71; value of examining, 57–59

Basic practice allowance, 35
Belgium, 25
Benchmarking, 12–13
Beveridge Report, 30
Breast cancer screening, 69–70
Burden of disease, ix, 13, 93–94, 97–101, 123; in U.S., x, 112
Business, privileged position of, 6

Caisse Nationale d'Assurance Maladie des Professions Indèpendants (CANAM), 31
Caisse Nationale d'Assurance Maladie des Travailleurs Salariés (CNAMTS), 31
Canada, 3, 14, 16, 23, 25, 36, 38, 80, 93, 113, 123; and Commonwealth Fund, 12
Capitated payments, 33
Cardiac catheterization, 18
Case studies, 1, 4
Centers for Disease Control and Prevention (CDC), 40, 58
Centers of medical excellence, 53
Chronic disease, 17, 30, 75–76
Clinical trials, 13
Commonwealth Fund, 12–13, 74; and International Working Group on Quality Indicators, 16
Comparative analysis, 1, 8; and adjusting for need, 113; of allocation of resources, 25; of health systems, 12; of high-tech innovations, 18; and OECD, 117; value of city-level, 3–7, 114, 116
Congestive heart failure, 17, 73, 74, 83, 96, 104
Consultants, 38
Contractual model, 26
Convergent trends, 47–48
Coronary Artery Bypass Graph (CABG) Surgery, 18, 93, 96, 104; gender disparities in, 110–111; need for, 113, 123
Council for Health Improvement, 38
Culture, 17, 39, 112, 119

Databases, 5; and OECD health, 8
Denmark, 15, 18, 24–25, 93
Deprivation, 5, 44, 63, 67; and avoidable hospital conditions, 83, 88; and avoidable mortality, 70; and revascularization, 104
Diabetes, 17, 24, 62, 65, 73, 74–76, 83
Diagnosis-related groupings (DRGs), 34, 36
Disability Adjusted Life Expectancy (DALE): and differences in use of resources, 10; and missing data, 9
Disease: burden of, ix–x, 13, 93–94, 97–101, 112, 123; chronic, 17, 30, 75–76
Disease surveillance, 46–47, 120–121. See also Syndromic surveillance
Disparities, viii–ix, 3; in access, 63, 71, 80; in AHCs, 18, 83; in avoidable mortality, 57, 59, 66–68, 71; between cities, 104–109; between countries, 79, 95, 122; ethnic, 109, 123; gender, 19, 59, 94, 109–112; in heart disease treatment, 109–112; in infant mortality, 48; in London, 43, 109; in Manhattan, ix, 85, 90, 115, 123; between neighborhoods, 47–48, 66–68, 79, 85; in revascularization, 94, 104–109

Electronic health records, 32
Epidemiological modeling, 14
Ethnicity, 18, 43; and barriers to primary care, 86–90, 124; and barriers to specialty care, 104–105, 109; and diversity in urban cores, 51–52; and primary care outcomes, 78
EuroBarometer, 9, 12
Europe, Western, 36
European Union Geriatric Medical Society (EUGMS), 58

Fee-for-service payments, 14, 33, 35, 37, 39, 45
Finland, 10
Fringe benefits, 26

Gender-adjusted rates, 56
General practitioners (GPs), 37, 38, 42, 43–44, 70; and payment for performance contracts, 76–78
General revenue, 22–23
Germany, 12
Global Cities, 7, 48; and command and control, 50
Globalization, 6–7; and health, 47–48, 75
Goals, 13
Government, 26; subnational, 3–4
Greece, 15
Guidelines, 35

Healthcare Resource Group (HRG), 36
Health maintenance organizations (HMOs), 36
Health needs, 7
Health services research, 3, 4, 116
Health status, 1, 23, 29, 42, 48, 52–53; and hospital use, 78, 81–83; and premature death, 56–57, 59, 70; and small area variation, 5–10
Hôpital Saint Louis, vii
Hospitals: investor-owned, 36; proprietary, 25; public, vii, 25

Ile de France, 47, 50
Immigrants, 39, 44, 116
Immunization, 45, 58, 81, 83, 151
Index, 18
Indicators, 7–8, 14, 17
Inequality, 3, 7, 50–51, 71, 85, 121, 125; in London, 42–43
Infant mortality, 14–15; reductions in, 16
Infrastructure, public health, viii, 19, 21; and city autonomy, 115
Inner cities, 5
Institute of Medicine, 29, 74
Insurance, 23–25, 28, 31, 33–34, 36, 69, 76, 77, 80, 82, 101, 103, 105–106, 112, 114, 122, 127; and access to care, 17–18; and AHCs, 85–86; for children, 27, 29, 39; employer-sponsored, 26–27; public, x; and tax deductibility, 22; universal, ix. See also National health insurance

International Association of Geriatrics and Gerontology (IAGG), 58
Inventory approach, 13
Ischemic heart disease (IHD), 93, 96–101; cross-national comparison of, 122; decline in rates of, 18; gender disparities in, 105, 109–112
Italy, 24

Japan, 10

Kerr-Mills Program, 27–28

Life expectancy, 13
London Development Agency, 42
London Health Commission, 42–43
Luxembourg, 25

Marker conditions, 82, 84, 91
McKinsey Global Institute, 16
Means test, 28
Medicaid, 27–29, 33, 39, 89–91, 105
Medical technology, 23
Medicare, 22, 27–29, 39, 74, 105; and DRGs, 34, 36; and fiscal intermediaries, 32; and resource-based relative value scale (RBRVS), 33
Megacities, 1–2, 118–119
Megapoles Project, 5, 119
Megatrend, 1
Memorial Sloan-Kettering Cancer Center, vii
Mobility of capital, 6; and global economic competition, 7
Mortality. *See* Avoidable mortality
Mutualité Sociale Agricole, 31

National Agency for Hospital Accreditation and Quality, 35
National Agency on Health Accreditation and Evaluation, 35
National Committee on Public Health, 35
National health insurance (NHI), 23, 25, 126; French system of, 29–32, 34–36; and physician payment, 45
National health policies, 19; and consequences for cities, 124–127

National Health Service (NHS), 23–26, 32–33, 35, 37–38, 41–44, 69–70, 76, 93, 95, 101, 109, 114, 126; and local authorities, 38, 43; and primary care trusts (PCT), 33, 35, 38, 42–44, 70, 76; and regional health authorities, 37–38; and strategic health authority, 41–43
National Institute for Health and Clinical Effectiveness (NICE), 38
National service frameworks, 32
Negative binomial regression, 63, 66–68
Neighborhoods, 2, 17
Netherlands, the, 12
New Labour, 38
New York City Department of Emergency Management, 40
New York City Department of Health and Mental Hygiene, 40, 48; and A1C registry, 41; and Citywide Colon Cancer Control Coalition, 41; and smoking ban, 41
New York City Health and Hospitals Corporation (HHC), 39–40, 45
New Zealand, 10, 12

Organization of Economic Cooperation and Development (OECD), 57, 93, 95, 123; and health database, 12; and health services research, 3, 8, 16, 78–79; and heart disease treatment, 18, 113; largest cities in, 6; and national health systems, 21–25, 36–37; and premature mortality, 14
Out-of-pocket payments, 23–24, 30, 101

Paris City Council, 45
Paris Department of Health and Social Action (DASES), 45–46
Percutaneous Transluminal Coronary Angioplasty (PTCA), 18, 110, 113, 123; factors that explain use of, 104; high rate of, in U.S., 93–94
Performance, 7–9, 13–16; high, 12; and mortality, 56–60; new approach to, 17; and outcomes, 121–124; published information on, 32–33; and rankings, 10–11; and responsiveness,

Performance *(cont.)*
11; universal criteria for, 11; WHO
ranking of, 37
Physicians: consultants, 38; general
practitioners (GPs), 37, 38, 42,
43–44, 70, 76–78; payment of, 45;
sector 1 and 2, 45; solo-based private
practice, 37
Pneumonia, 17, 62, 74, 83
Point of service (POS) plans, 36
Policies, national, 19; and consequences
for cities, 124–127
Policy learning, 1–2
Political culture, 17, 112
Politique de Ville, 48–49
Population density, 50, 53
Potential Years of Life Lost, 11, 18
Poverty, vii, 3, 29, 39, 85, 91; as urban
core characteristic, 50–51
Practice styles, 5
Preferred provider organizations
(PPOs), 36
Premature mortality, 15
Prenatal care, 2
Presbyterian Medical Center, vii
Prevention, 13; primary, 71; secondary
41, 58, 62, 69, 121
Primary care, 7, 12–13, 32, 37–38,
39–40, 70, 74–76, 122; appropriate,
18; and better outcomes, 78–79;
definition of, 77–78; measurement
of, 78–81
Primary care trusts, 38, 70, 76; and
gatekeepers, 42; and health equity
audits, 43; and London Strategic
Health Authority, 43
Production function approach, 14
Progressivity, 12
Public health infrastructure, viii, 19, 21;
and city autonomy, 115
Public opinion, 9

Quasi-public organizations, 31

Race, 18, 52, 67, 114; as barrier to
primary care, 86, 88, 89–91; as
barrier to specialty care, 103,
104–106, 109; and geographic
concentration of poverty, 123

Rates, gender-adjusted, 56
Rationing, 30
Regression analysis, 15
Research, health services, 3, 4,
116
Revascularization, ix, 18–19, 69;
and access to specialty care,
122–123; disparities in, 104–109;
and low-income arrondissements,
114; national comparisons of,
93–95; ratio of, to AMI, 102

Safety-net, health care, 4, 17, 29, 39,
45, 80, 91, 124
Sector 1 and 2 physicians, 45
Social Security, 12, 22, 25, 31, 35; and
amendments of 1965, 27
Solo-based private practice physicians, 37
Spain, 24
Specialists, 37, 39, 42, 53, 77
Spending, 21, 30
State Child Health Insurance Program
(SCHIP), 27, 29, 39
Subnational government, 3–4
Suburbs, 2
Sweden, 10
Switzerland, 23, 79
Syndromic surveillance, 40–41

Tax, payroll, 23, 25
Tokyo, 6, 118
Trends, convergent, 47–48
Tuberculosis, 17, 40, 70,
118–119

Uninsured people, 22, 81, 91, 105
United Nations, 1, 49–50, 117
Universal coverage, vii; and
government-run systems, x; and
universal health insurance, ix
Urban cores, viii, 6, 19, 80, 90,
93–94, 97, 101, 109, 121, 123,
127; as unit of analysis, 49–54
Urban health penalty, 2, 118–119;
and contradictory evidence, 120
Urban studies, 4

Values, 9
Variations, small-area, 5

Veterans Health Administration, 37, 39
Vulnerable populations, 3

Waiting lists, 38
Welfare policies, 7; and U.S. as welfare laggard, 8
Welfare state, 4, 8, 46, 116, 125
Western Europe, 36

Women's health, 14; and avoidable hospital conditions, 91; and gender disparities, 19; and mortality, 15; and revascularization, 109–112
World cities, vii, 55
World Health Organization (WHO), 9–13, 58; and healthy cities project, 5, 42; and millennium report, 29; and MONICA Project, 95–96
World War II, 24, 46

MICHAEL K. GUSMANO, PH.D., is a research scholar at the Hastings Center in Garrison, New York. He is also the co-director of the World Cities Project (WCP) at the International Longevity Center–USA (ILC-USA), in New York City. He is the author of *Healthy Voices/Unhealthy Silence: Advocating for Poor People's Health* (with Colleen Grogan), co-author and editor of *Growing Older in World Cities: New York, London, Paris, and Tokyo* (with Victor Rodwin), and author of more than 50 journal articles and reports. He holds a Ph.D. in political science from the University of Maryland at College Park, earned a master's in public policy from the State University of New York at Albany, and was a postdoctoral fellow at Yale University.

VICTOR G. RODWIN, M.P.H., PH.D., is a professor of health policy and management in the Robert Wagner School of Public Service at New York University, in New York. With Dr. Gusmano, he is the co-director of the WCP. He is author and editor of many books, including *The Health Planning Predicament: France, Québec, England, and the United States; The End of an Illusion: The Future of Health Policy in Western Industrialized Nations* (with J. de Kervasdoué and J. Kimberly); *Public Hospital Systems in New York City and Paris* (with D. Jolly, C. Brecher, and R. Banter); *Growing Older in World Cities: New York, London, Paris, and Tokyo* (with Michael Gusmano); and most recently, *Universal Health Insurance in France: Is It Sustainable?* He has a B.A. in economics from the University of Wisconsin and received a master's degree in public health and a Ph.D. in city and regional planning, both from the University of California, Berkeley.

DANIEL WEISZ, M.D., M.P.A., a former thoracic surgeon, is a senior research associate with the WCP. From 1982 to 1999, he was an attending surgeon in cardiothoracic surgery at St. Francis Hospital, Roslyn, New York, and assistant clinical professor of cardiothoracic surgery at the Albert Einstein College of Medicine. Before joining

St. Francis Hospital, from 1975 to 1982 he was a staff surgeon in cardiothoracic surgery at Long Island Jewish–Hillside Medical Center, New Hyde Park, New York, and assistant professor of surgery at SUNY Stony Brook. Dr. Weisz received his M.D. from Johns Hopkins University School of Medicine and his M.P.A. in health policy and management from New York University's Wagner School. Before joining the ILC-USA in 2001, Dr. Weisz was a fellow with the minority staff of the Health Subcommittee of the Ways and Means Committee, U.S. House of Representatives.